Praise for *Building a Better Boomer*

"Neil Offen has become one of America's greatest humorists, embracing the lighter side of the aging process with charm and wit culled from personal experience. His columns, and now this book, have become must-read."

—**Marty Appel**, *New York Times* bestselling author of *Pinstripe Empire* and *Munson*

"Neil Offen's timing is perfect. This is the moment when we need a book that is this funny—Offen makes us laugh at subjects that are not supposed to be funny, which may be the definition of the best humor. *Building a Better Boomer* never stops and never misfires."

—**Mark Kurlansky**, *New York Times* bestselling author of *Salt; Cod;* and *The Importance of Not Being Ernest*

"Neil Offen offers laugh-out-loud—but still practical—advice about how to deal with the indignities of growing older, all the while trying to combat aging and aging stereotypes. This is a book for all boomers, and those who care for and love them."

—**Steven Petrow**, contributing columnist *The Washington Post* and author, *Stupid Things I Won't Do When I Get Old*

"I have often heard it said that there is nothing funny about growing older. Well, as Neil Offen proves—hysterically—in *Building a Better Boomer,* that is wildly inaccurate. If laughter truly is the best medicine, this is a book that I heartily prescribe for my fellow boomers. Offen's sharp—and unfortunately accurate—observations will make you laugh out loud, assuming of course you can remember where you left your reading glasses. Let me suggest that the nicest thing you can give to one of our peers is this gift of laughter."

— **David Fisher**, *New York Times* bestselling author

"There's no better source of smiles, laughs, even guffaws, as your body deteriorates and your role in society diminishes, than these essays by humor-writer-nonpareil Neil Offen."

—**Mitchell Stephens**, author of *The Voice of America: Lowell Thomas and the Invention of 20th-Century Journalism*

"Neil Offen's hilarious *Building a Better Boomer* is a rare mix of laugh-out-loud and close-to-the-bone. Sure, it's funny but it's also insightful, sweet, and even provocative. You will read this book to laugh and keep from crying, because, as Neil so shrewdly observes, 'there is a limit on how much better we can become.'"

—**Frank Van Riper**, author of *Recovered Memory: New York & Paris 1960-1980*

"This is a great book. I know that because my husband, Neil Offen, told me so. (Also, he threatened to take away my top billing in the Acknowledgments if I didn't write this.)"

—**Carol Offen** (no relation to this book's author other than by marriage)

Building a Better Boomer

Building a Better Boomer

How to deal with bothersome bodies, exhausting exercise, memory missteps, terrifying technology, impossible insurance, retirement regrets, foreign foods, and, oh yeah, aging

Neil Offen

Paperback ISBN 13: 978-1-08-790-860-1
E-book ISBN 13: 978-1-08-791-129-8
First Edition 2023

For Carol, Paul, and Nora,
who have put up with me since carbon paper days.

Contents

Aging: It's Not for Everyone 1

Building a Better Body

The reign of pain 9
Dealing with it 13
Keeping an eye out 16
Falling into place 20

Building a Better Brain

A mind is a terrible thing 27
Forget about it 30
Achieving perfect recall 33
Don't forget about it 37

Building a Better Patient

What's up, doc? 43
Side-by-side effects 48
In case of emergency 52
Caring about Medicare 56
Choose your coverage 61

Building a Better Build

The shape of things 67
Exercising our demons 70
How to get started 73
Witness to fitness 76
Work those quads! 80
Run for your life 84
Last lap 88

Building a Better Sleeper

Losing our snoozing 93
Dreaming of dozing 97
Napping for dummies 102

Building a Better Diet

Food for thought 107
The nutrition condition 110
What you should eat 114
Weight, weight, don't tell me 118

→ *Update Alert* ← 122

Building a Better Techie

Digital overload 129
Between two worlds 134
What's the word? 138
Call for security 143
Terms of endearment 146
Anti-Social 149
Ask Mr. Techie 153

Building a Better Retirement

Is there life after work? 161
Laying the groundwork 164
Money matters 166
What makes a good retirement? 173
Together forever 178
You've got (to have) a friend 181

Frequently Asked Questions 186
In Closing 191
Acknowledgments 194
About the Author 197
Index 200

Aging: It's Not for Everyone

Is sixty-five truly the new forty-five? Or could it be the new fifty in a certain kind of less-flattering light? On the other hand, wouldn't all of us baby boomers really rather be the old forty-five or even fifty and not just plain, you know, old?

But here most of us are: gray haired, stiff backed, and still using a Hotmail email address, and we need to come to grips with the truth, as difficult as that may be. It's difficult because many of us boomers not only don't consider ourselves old, we keep trying so hard to be younger, even occasionally wistfully watching *High School Musical 3: Senior Year*. We are a generation lost in space (for those who don't remember, that's "American Pie," by Don McLean, born just three months too soon to be an official baby boomer).

It doesn't matter if we can do several sets of burpees and check our ECG results on our Apple Watch. We still can't think of ourselves as "with it," particularly since no one under the age of fifty says "with it" anymore. The harsh reality is that movies and television still want us off their screens. Businesses want us off their payrolls. Our children want us off the dance floor.

Yes, TV commercials may occasionally use *our* music, from the fifties, sixties, and seventies, but the people partying and dancing and drinking beer on the beach are clearly not us. They have more hair, their skin is smoother despite being covered by tattoos, and they almost never call out that they've fallen and can't get up.

We, on the other hand, are the ones in the occasional commercial for bladder control medications, Medicare supplement plans, and a drug—who knows what it does?—called Taltz (rhymes with *schmaltz*).

After screwing up the world for the last fifty years or so, baby boomers are clearly no longer lead players in our culture (except in government, of course). We have become generic character actors, comic relief, like Chester in *Gunsmoke*, a reference surely lost on people busy streaming *Stranger Things* and *White Lotus* and debating the end of *Succession*. We boomers rightly sense we may have become irrelevant to the central story, unconnected to the moment's gestalt, which many of us believe may be a digestive disorder.

Is it surprising, then, that we have become the butt of "ok, boomer" jokes? Yes, admittedly, we have ruined the planet, despoiled the oceans, and bear much of the responsibility for the success of *Celebrity Apprentice*. But does all that justify becoming the coronavirus's target demographic, constantly referred to as the elderly, the fragile, the at-risk, and worst of all, the dead?

Not that long ago—when older people were just called old people before the word *seniors* was invented—age and maturity were revered. Youth was something to grow out of, like tie-dyed pants and Nehru jackets.

Older generations consequently weren't obsessed with staying young forever. They were content to watch the world pass them by. They knew they had wisdom, perspective, and 5 percent off on senior day at the supermarket. They were okay with slowly fading away, as long as they could do it from their La-Z-Boy recliners.

Boomers, not so much.

No longer young, many of us continue wanting to *seem* young, trying to act young. And it's not easy.

Inundated with how-to-stay-healthy advice, we use anti-aging face cream and regenerative moisturizer (SPF 132!) and drink bottled water from pristine springs rather than Mello Yello from God knows where. We eliminate gluten from our diet and try ingesting more antioxidants and fewer oxidants, if we could figure out which are which.

We hire a personal trainer, then check our target heart rate on a Fitbit as if we understood what's a target heart rate. We play pickleball and are disappointed to learn no gherkins are involved. We go to yoga and Pilates and Zumba and Tai Chi and would do downward dog if we could figure out how to do upward dog immediately afterward.

We play brain games to ward off dementia and do Qi

Gong to ward off osteoporosis. We get new knees, replace our hips, and swap out our rotator cuffs.

Awash in unfamiliar popular culture, we nevertheless think we can distinguish between Dua Lipa and Doja Cat before recognizing we have no idea who either of them is. We have a bunch of Spotify and Pandora playlists but also a stack of old 45s, Guess Who cassette tapes, and three nonambulatory Walkmans. We like to imagine we'd get all the references in *Saturday Night Live* skits, but of course we never watch it live because it's on too late.

At sea in a high-tech storm, we Zoom with friends, Skype with former colleagues, and WhatsApp with family but still don't know how to find those digital photos from that trip to Greece. We're finally on Instagram when everyone has migrated over to TikTok. We now have so many gizmos and a bounty of complex thingamajigs, along with several completely unnecessary doohickeys, but still can't figure out how the QR code works. And when something goes wrong with our iPhone 32, we have to find a nearby twelve-year-old to fix it.

We do all this trying to hold on to our youthful past, but it's hard, especially when our past happened back before we were paying attention. Plus, when you get older, there's a lot more past to remember. And now there's a lot more complicated present to deal with.

In addition to the traditional problems involved with getting older—increasing bodily frailty, faulty memory, root canals—our generation also confronts some unique challenges, including maple almond butter Snickers bars, mounting

LinkedIn requests from people we've never heard of, and receiving mail with an invitation to a complimentary dinner where you can learn about cremation (I chose the salmon entrée.).

We find ourselves living in a world where the print size of menus seems to have become smaller and restaurants appear to have become catastrophically louder, and frequently we feel much less capable of dealing with it all, particularly if there are acronyms involved. How do we navigate this scary world and make believe we really understand text messages that end with KMN? (I looked it up; it's Kill Me Now.)

But FIHNI. (Frankly, I Have No Idea.)

HIGTTTSYHTA (However, I'm going to try to show you how to anyway.)

Building a Better Body

The reign of pain

The sobering news: Each year past the age of forty we lose 3.5 percent of our muscle mass. Without that extra muscle mass, we sometimes find that performing difficult physical activities, like bending down to tie our shoes, causes us pain. We can get winded when we go for a brisk walk to the bathroom at 3 a.m. We may find it hard to lift heavy objects, like our arms.

Getting up from a chair can be daunting, particularly if we've been there for the entire *Cheers* TV rerun marathon. Opening a can of soup, a major test of physical prowess, can be next to impossible, particularly if it has one of those rigid easy-open metal tabs, which are always rigid but never easy.

We can feel the loss of muscle mass all the way from flabby ear lobes to sagging arches. With less muscle mass, our backs have gotten stiffer and our knees have gotten creakier. Pretty much everything has started to ache.

The other morning, for instance, when I woke up—always good news—there was a painful crick in my neck. This was not, I must admit, wholly unexpected, since aren't we at the age when something cricks almost every morning when we get up?

When I turned my head to back the car out of the driveway later that morning, there was this sharp, snapping sound, and I'm reasonably certain it wasn't the side-view mirror once again hitting the side of the garage door.

The crick led to a shooting pain at the side of my head, and to maneuver my neck back to where it normally belonged, I twisted my shoulder, felt a popping in my spine, hurt my knee when I tried to straighten my back, and stubbed my foot when I straightened my knee. All in all, annoyingly typical for a man my age who is in excellent health for someone 132 years old.

These aches and pains, we realize, are our new normal. Today the right hip seems out of joint. Tomorrow it may be the left shoulder that throbs. Last week it was definitely that new mysterious thump in the chest. And it's *always* the knees. You remember when the left knee gave out, walking down the stairs? And two weeks ago, walking up the stairs, wasn't it the right knee that suddenly made that ominous scraping sound?

Depending on the day, there are, for almost all boomers, a number of intermittent aches, pains, twinges, cramps, pangs, stitches, stabs, spasms, pinches, stings, and otherwise unidentified throbbing sensations. Sometimes, inconveniently, a body part falls off.

Let's be clear: Most of the time, none of these aches and

pains is a particularly big deal. At least for the moment. Like many of us, I am generally healthy and, in fact, I believe, quite normal for my age. The problem is my age.

Despite all our efforts, our once reasonably robust baby boomer physiques seem to be deteriorating just a little bit more with each passing hour, particularly if that hour is spent chewing on Cheetos. With every year, our waistlines are expanding, our spines are contracting, our hair is receding, plus there are also some really very irritating paper cuts.

In fact, if we're honest with ourselves, we know our lifetime warranty may be nearing expiration. Worse, it apparently won't cover any damage to the product caused by smoking back when we were in college because we all thought, at the time, smoking looked cool. Nor does it cover intentional misuse, such as Twinkies. It doesn't include discs that are slipping or rotator cuffs that no longer rotate. Defects in materials and workmanship—nope, not covered either.

According to many younger researchers who have never been troubled by random heart palpitations, the mitochondria in our cells, the building blocks of other building blocks, weaken as we age. They split apart and sometimes begin scattering all over the kitchen floor. Frequently, these aimless little mitochondria can roll helplessly into corners under the dishwasher where you can't reach them without bending all the way down and who wants to bend all the way down if you then have to bend all the way up again, given the dizziness potential?

Numerous studies have shown that, as we all know, mitochondrial deterioration contributes to cellular senescence, chronic inflammation, a decline in stem cell activity, and general crankiness when you are disturbed during a nap.

And here's the really bad news: according to reports from the National Academy of Perpetual Doomsayers, further mitochondrial deterioration is forecast for the future, along with potentially gusty winds; and torrential aches and pains, maybe even bunions, are likely to arise. These signs of physical decline will become as regular as we no longer are.

Unless . . .

Dealing with it

SURE, GIVEN THE ALTERNATIVE, NEW ACHES AND PAINS are the price we are willing to pay for still being alive, even when there's nothing good that's new on Netflix.

But that means we need to confront the depressing reality that our bunions now have corns, our shoulders can no longer shoulder the burden, reflux keeps returning, and we have begun babbling so much about our various aches and pains that our friends will interrupt us to talk about *anything* else, even Congress.

In other words, we need to find a way to live with our increasing bodily deterioration—and remind ourselves that the twinge in the calf or the throb in the shoulder is, for the moment, nothing more than a twinge in the calf or a throb in the shoulder (until, of course, it isn't).

That is, it's all really a question of perspective. Here's what I mean:

Look on the bright side. When you get a cramp in your foot and can't walk, remember you most likely have another foot. Let it work for its keep! It may turn out that this foot was your favorite one all along.

Don't fight it. If your back is so stiff you can't stand up after sitting for hours on the couch, then don't. Stay on the couch. It's likely that another episode of *Two and a Half Men* will be coming on shortly.

Hold tight to the past. When your shoulder aches and you can't lift your arm up above your head, remember yesterday when your head ached and you were able to completely ignore your shoulder.

Find a quick fix. If you feel a tingling sensation at your fingertips, let go of the ice cream and close the freezer.

Ignore. Don't pay any attention to the relentless clicking of your hip or the extreme tenderness in your elbow. You will soon forget all about them during your colonoscopy prep.

Fight the power. While it's rarely a good sign to hear yourself gasping for breath when you are exercising, or particularly when you are scrambling eggs, turn up the volume in your headphones or hearing aids and drown it out.

Consider alternatives. If you frequently get a crick in the neck while turning your head all the way to the right when backing the car out of the driveway, turn your head all the way to the left or leave the car in the driveway. Hail a taxi. Call an Uber. Hitchhike down the road. Or go back inside to watch TV and hope that something other than *Two and a Half Men* is on.

Slow down and relax. Instead of worrying too much

about that pounding sensation in your chest and the growing paralysis of your right hand, take a moment to meditate. Sit down, mindfully settle into your place, notice the sounds around you, gently focus on the breath, and then, in your own time, call for the ambulance.

Keeping an eye out

For me, as for many, the eyes went first. Even back in elementary school, I needed to cheat on the eye test.

It was a victimless crime, if you don't count the ophthalmologist, who lost a number of co-pays. As other kids would stand in the back of the classroom, cover an eye, and read from the chart placed at the front of the classroom, I'd memorize what they'd recite: Z F G H S D, and so on. So, when it came to my turn, no one would know that I was so nearsighted I could only see the Z and thought it was an S. Or maybe an H. How about a $?

(Also, to be frank, I had no idea what ZFGHSD meant, although I thought it could have been a Serbo-Croatian acronym for ophthalmologist.)

Like many of us did, I cheated because I didn't want to wear contact lenses, which had not yet been invented, nor glasses, which had been expressly invented to make nine-year-old boys look almost as dorky as using a pen protector, soon to be banned by the Geneva Conventions. And like many nine-year-old boys of our generation, I also thought wearing glasses would complicate my career plan of playing centerfield for the Yankees. Professional ballplayers didn't wear glasses. Or, for that matter, pocket pen protectors.

Even then I understood that my eyesight wasn't great and I should have acknowledged my problem and gotten help for it. But like many of us, particularly many of us now, I was willing to bump into walls occasionally as long as I wouldn't have to admit I couldn't see those walls right in front of me.

Unfortunately, as we get older, our eyesight generally doesn't improve (unless we have cataract surgery and suddenly can see that we've been wearing mismatched socks for the last nine years).

Like many boomers, I now have increased difficulty reading the fine print and even the not-so-fine print, meaning I have no idea why Capital One has recently updated its terms of service and privacy policy. The print on restaurant menus, deviously designed by millennials in an attempt to dominate the printer-to-table menu market, is now so minute we are forced to order only entrées and have to forgo appetizers, side dishes, and worse, sometimes dessert. Movie subtitles in English look like they might be in French. Stop signs along the road appear to say *top*.

And most important, there's no longer an opportunity to memorize what my sixth-grade comrade Phyllis Levine's perfect eyesight had revealed. Meaning the only thing that's clear now is the obvious: that we can no longer fool anyone, even ourselves, into thinking that we can see clearly.

How, then, can we compensate for the natural diminution of our eyesight even if we are reluctant to admit there's been a natural diminution of our eyesight?

Here are some possibilities:

Buy a larger TV. If the 256-inch set that has taken over your entire living room is starting to seem insufficient, and you can barely make out Vin Diesel's facial features while you stream *Fast & Furious* 26, get the new 514-inch model, which can take over your breakfast nook as well. To pay for the set, charge family members for the popcorn. And also recognize that Vin Diesel may not have any facial features.

Use your other senses more. When you are driving at night on a desolate mountain road, smell where the next blind turn will be. If that doesn't work, listen carefully for the sound of yourself screaming, "what the hell am I doing on a desolate mountain road in the middle of the night?"

Increase the lighting in your home. Get rid of all those 100-watt bulbs and even the squiggly 16-watt equivalents and replace them with the arc lights from left field at Fenway Park. Be sure to get a dimmer switch, too.

Walk with your arms thrust out in front of you. Remember, it's always possible there's a wall nearby.

Move your laptop. It can sometimes be difficult to see what's on your computer screen when your eyesight is no longer 20/20 and the years have moved on quite a bit from 2020. But despite its name, a laptop does not have to go on your lap. You can move it up to your chest or even your neck, much closer to your eyes, while you also increase the font size on your screen to Times New Roman 786 (equivalent to Calibri 1088).

Employ contrast. You want to make things you can't see clearly stand out as much as possible. So put milk in a dark coffee cup or put colored bright strips on the edge of dark stairs or put a dab of hot fudge sundae sauce on your new white shirt. Then you can tell everyone you did it on purpose.

Reduce glare. Pull down the shades and close the curtains. You won't be able to see any better, but at least none of your neighbors will be able to see you stumbling around and banging your head on the refrigerator.

Use magnification. Take a small problem and make it bigger by ignoring it.

Falling into place

Then there's falling. As we age, it happens more frequently and can have serious consequences. Like not getting up.

Along with many in our age group, I have some experience with falling. I have fallen walking down steps; I have fallen walking up steps; I also have fallen on escalator steps, both going down and going up, and on moving walkways at airports, going nowhere at all.

(Once, during a recent 5K race I ran, I even fell twice. The other runners were very solicitous as they raced past me each time after I fell, carefully avoiding the blood and being sure not to step on me, which might slow them down. And if you're wondering why I was running a 5K race in the first place, it's because there were no 1Ks around and my wife wanted to declutter the pantry.)

Falling is serious business when you get to your sixties and seventies. As we are constantly reminded, in 87 percent of cases in people sixty-five and over, falls are the number-one cause of people landing on the ground. The risk of falling increases proportionately with age. At eighty years, more than half of seniors fall annually, usually sometime in December if they want to beat the end-of-year deadline.

Because we are supposedly less agile and more fragile, falls can lead to a broken hip or at the very least people stepping over you when they are hurrying to catch the 5:06 to Greenwich. Falls can reduce your mobility and damage your credibility with your personal trainer. They are also the leading cause of injury and the second leading cause of extreme embarrassment among seniors, just behind arriving too late for restaurants' early bird specials. A fall can be particularly embarrassing when it happens if you are just brushing your teeth or when you are bragging to your children about how age hasn't slowed you down.

Falling is generally a question of balance. Like many of us, I haven't any. When I stand up too quickly after sitting for too long on the couch, I frequently lose my balance. If I try to find it, I get light-headed and trip over the couch. When I do find it, I still trip over the couch. My balance is so limited I cannot stand on one foot while trying to put my other foot into my pants. I am considering sitting down while putting on my pants or wearing kilts.

Most falls, of course, occur in the home, where we are more likely to fall because we haven't been out of the home much since three years ago March. But some falls occur outside, in public places, like big-box stores, where you are less likely to be able to blame your partner, who never left home.

How can we prevent falls and, if we do fall, how can we avoid the worst consequences, like being surreptitiously videotaped and shared as a GIF on some young clown's Instagram account? Here are a few tips:

Practice mindfulness. Focus on the present and be aware of your surroundings, instead of being lost in your thoughts. This way, if you start to fall, you will definitely know it and have time to prepare an excuse and to figure out who in your household you can blame.

Take smaller steps while walking. Long strides are more difficult to control, so think short and mincing. It may take you longer to get where you are going, but it might also get you into a Broadway chorus line.

Scan the path ahead of you. Notice if there are any obstacles in your way, like buildings. Check for sinkholes in the pavement. Though you may not find any, by checking you could pick up a few pennies along the way, though you might also accidentally blunder into dog poop or the high-occupancy lane of an interstate.

Avoid carrying items that might block your ability to see the ground in front of you. The added benefit is that you can get your spouse to shlep the groceries from the car while you drink a negroni.

Fall-proof your house. Put hand rails on all sides of the living room, including the fireplace. Remove all furniture from the bedroom. Sleep on the floor so if you fall when getting up it's not from a great height. Don't leave tripping hazards—like shoes, purses, and the refrigerator—on the floor, particularly in areas where you commonly walk. Keep your house brightly lit so you will be able to see the coffee table you trip over. Secure loose rugs by hammering them onto the wall. Avoid standing on chairs or stools while running. Instead of using a step stool, become taller. Use grab bars and a nonslip mat in the shower, and then super glue your feet to the mat. Better yet, just use hand sanitizer to clean your entire body.

Check your footwear. You don't want to flip, which frequently leads to a flop, so attach external traction cleats to your flip-flops. Though this may leave some marks in your wall-to-wall carpeting, you can use your slip-resistant cleats to scratch behind your ears if you are double-jointed. If you are not, you can use them to scratch behind somebody else's ears.

Be extra careful going up or down stairs. If your stairs are particularly steep, consider installing a zip line. If there are just a few steps, ask a neighbor to carry you.

If you start to fall, try to stay relaxed. The stiffer you are, the more likely an injury. So, while falling, think of a tranquil beach vacation in Cancun. Remember the joy of taking the last french fry when your partner wasn't looking. Hum "Here Comes the Sun" even if you can't recall the words.

Don't stick out your hands. When falling forward, the natural instinct is to stick out your hands to break the impact, thereby breaking your wrists instead. If possible, try to land on your side or at least on someone's side. If that's not possible, bring your hands together and try to pray, very quickly.

Try to avoid hitting your head. If you are falling backward, tuck your chin to your chest, round your back, pull your knees up to your diaphragm and curse all the fall-prevention advice that recommends you do all that in the split second you are falling.

Building a Better Brain

A mind is a terrible thing

As the pains and aches and falls accumulate, do you sometimes think you're also losing your mind? This is not uncommon, particularly at a certain age. According to the federal Bureau of Lost and Found, nearly 6.2 million minds have been lost over the last decade, many of which did not have names sewn on the back or printed on the collar in magic marker.

In fact, many of us boomers, worried about the possibility of incipient dementia, have lost our minds over worrying about simple problems like losing our keys. We think, perhaps with some validity, that this may be the beginning of an irreversible slide into musing about the first time we heard the Beatles as well as, inevitably, increased drooling.

When we can't find our glasses or remember who was our high school prom date or the names of our children, we naturally start to think we are on the precipice of cognitive decline.

But let's be honest: if we were really on the precipice of cognitive decline, would we actually use a phrase like "the precipice of cognitive decline"? And doesn't everybody lose keys occasionally and misplace glasses, although, admittedly, not usually on the middle rack of the oven?

Not every forgetful moment means Alzheimer's is knocking at the door. It could instead just be pinging you with a text or inviting you to a Zoom. But that doesn't mean we shouldn't be aware of the real signs of the possible beginnings of truly losing our minds. Here's how to tell:

Have you had episodes of short-term memory loss? For instance, do you sometimes forget why you got in the shower? If you think it was to go to the movies, you may have a problem unless you can remember if there was a second feature or at least twenty minutes of previews of movies you'll never want to see. (Additional advice: never order popcorn while in the shower.)

Do you have trouble communicating? Can you explain to friends and family the plot of *The Crown*? Can you describe, in detail, the relationship of Margaret, Countess of Snowdon, to Wallis, Duchess of Windsor? Do your friends and family have no idea what you're talking about because they've been watching *Wipeout* on TBS?

Are you occasionally confused? When you're in the self-checkout line at the supermarket, are you puzzled about what code to put in for loose donuts and whether that is different from the code for pastries? And are you puzzled about whether croissants are also considered pastries? Relax, everybody is puzzled by croissants, except the French.

Are you frequently moody? It's okay to be depressed about whether you are pronouncing croissants correctly and then immediately elated about knowing it's donuts and no longer doughnuts.

Have you developed an inability to grasp sarcasm? Yeah, right, of course you haven't.

Do you have difficulty performing simple tasks? You've just done the laundry and now all you have to do is fold the fitted sheet. And then refold the fitted sheet. And then throw the damn sucker out the window.

Do you occasionally have bouts of confusion? Do you still have no idea who Olivia Rodrigo is? Matty Healy? The Weeknd? Mitch McConnell? Can you not figure out which remote is for the TV, which one for the DVD player, and which one for the VCR — and why do you still have a VCR? Are you overwhelmed by how many Cheerio flavors are now available? (Stick with Honey Oat.)

Have you experienced a lack of interest in pretty much everything? No longer absorbed by the activities you used to enjoy, such as solo space travel and ultramarathon sledding? This is probably normal, but you should nevertheless get it checked out, preferably before the next time you board a rocket.

Do you have problems coping? Do you fall apart, melt into tears, or fly into a rage when you are unable to open a flip-top can of corn because the flip-top just broke off?

Join the club.

Forget about it

Okay, we can admit that occasionally we can't remember stuff: where we put the house keys, if we left the water running in the bathtub or the Pythagorean theorem. Maybe our spouse's name. Yes, this happens to all of us from time to time. In fact, studies show that about a third of healthy older adults have trouble knowing where I put my glasses.

It's a normal part of aging, a function of the brain, having been operating on high for a number of decades, now overloaded with useless information like who was Michael Dukakis's running mate in 1988 (Lloyd Bentsen) and the last line of the movie *Some Like It Hot* ("Nobody's perfect," of course.).

According to the most recent research, when we reach the age of forty or so, every minute of the day we start losing 17,211 brain cells, and even more if we're watching a Republican presidential debate. And the remaining cells have to work extra hard and so really get winded, forcing the cerebellum to just want to lie down on the couch and take a nap. Plus, with so many brain cells gone, it's naturally tough to remember where you put the car keys, even if you put them in the ignition.

And yet, though we occasionally forget the word for that large African animal with tusks and a trunk, we do remember odd bits of fluff. For instance, I can immediately sing along to all the words from Little Richard's "You Keep A-Knocking, But You Can't Come In" (admittedly, the song has only about eleven words, and they are repeated multiple times, but still), and I can recall, with little effort, the lineup of the 1960 Yankees.

But I managed to leave the house the other day without remembering to take my wallet. And it was not an isolated incident. On other occasions, I have forgotten my sunglasses while I was wearing them, didn't know where my cell phone was when talking on my cell phone with the store where I thought I had left my sunglasses, and walked into the kitchen to do something and then had no idea why I had walked into the kitchen, so walked into the living room and didn't understand why the refrigerator wasn't there.

Like all of us, I sometimes don't remember where I've put my slippers, my toothbrush, the mail I was carrying in from the mailbox, the newspaper I was just reading, or the cookie I was just sneaking. I've lost track of the joke I was telling, the conversation I was having and the lasagna I was baking.

I've also sometimes started sentences and forgotten midway through how they were supposed to . . .

(got it!) end.

We joke about these kind of memory lapses and call them "senior moments," mainly because we would rather not call them dementia. As we age and forget little things, and then more little things, we all start to develop a fear of dementia, which has polled badly and has a generally pejorative connotation. Every time we forget an inconsequential little thing—like, where are my keys? or what's the name of that actor in that show that we saw last night? or where do I live and who am I married to?—we understandably view it as a possible sign of incipient dementia.

My friend Marsha had exactly this fear a while ago. She had been forgetting things, like her glasses and where she parked her car, so she went to her doctor to ask for some tests to see if she might have early-onset Alzheimer's. The doctor reassured her that she was too old for early-onset anything.

Unfortunately, Marsha has no memory of the doctor appointment and still can't find her car. I, fortunately, have a garage.

Achieving perfect recall

The good news is there are ways to compensate for these senior moments.

Repeat what you want to remember. Say it several times silently to yourself. Or say it aloud as long as you are not in a crowded elevator and trying to remember the results of your urinalysis.

Write down things you need to remember. This can be a long list if you still care or a short list if you're retired and really don't give a damn. It can include occasionally hard-to-remember items like, "Get gas before the idiot light goes on, idiot" or vaguer but still important items like "Get up in the morning."

According to clinical trials of people who were forbidden the use of emojis to express themselves, it's preferable to actually write out by hand the things you want to remember, even if you need to write them in a cursive script that you can no longer decipher. This is preferable to jotting down what you want to remember on your smartphone, and then trying to figure out if you put those notes in notes, reminders, utilities, emails, texts, files, tips, Facebook or in Google Maps under favorite places.

Develop mnemonic devices. A mnemonic device is a kind of mnemory aid. The term is derived from the ancient Greek, *mnēmonikos*, which means, if I'm recalling correctly, carburetor. Mnemonic devices are, essentially, shortcuts—such as a rhyme, a saying, or an acronym—that will, you hope, remind you of the stuff you have forgotten.

Although you may not know the term, you probably have been using mnemonic devices for a long time. I have been using them since the seventh grade, which is why I still can tell you what the trigonometric functions are. [I know no one really cares, but in case my seventh-grade trig teacher is reading, it's Soak Your Toe. That is, SOH-CAH-TOA, which stands for Sine equals Opposite over Hypotenuse, Cosine equals Adjacent over Hypotenuse and Tangent equals Opposite Over Adjacent. And yeah, I have no idea what any of that means either.]

Roy G. Biv, for example, is how some of us remember the colors of the rainbow: red, orange, yellow, green, blue, indigo, and that other one. Then there's My Very Excellent Mother Just Served Us Nine Pizzas, which is a mnemonic device for remembering the order of the planets from the sun, if you ever receive a phone call asking you to list the names of the planets from the sun to win a $25 Amazon gift card.

There are lots of others, including ones for the Marine

Corps Guidelines for Machine Gun Emplacement, in case that comes in handy, the wives of Henry VIII, in chronological order, and the fate of the wives of Henry VIII, also in chronological order.

My wife has been using mnemonic devices for years, particularly when leaving the house, to make sure she has all of her stuff with her. Standing at the garage door, she recites a nonsense phrase she has created:

"Poor [phone] little [lunch] men [mask] play [pills] silly [sunglasses] dopey [drops, eye] kids' [keys] games [glasses] before [bag] Halloween [hearing aid] treats [tissues]," before walking out the door, getting in the car, and realizing she has forgotten to put on her shoes.

So, you can do this, too, to help you remember things. For instance, if you want to remember the names of all the No. 1 hits by the Beatles, take the first letter of each song and make it into an easy to remember phrase, like PFFTWVEFGBRYJZKD. It may help to hum it.

Create to-do lists. I have one right on my desk now. Some of the items on it date back to the late twentieth century. All the others, of course, are old.

There is no greater joy than crossing out an item that has been on your to-do list, even if you just put it on your to-do list after you just did it, simply so you could have the joy of crossing it out.

Use memory tools such as calendars. We have, for instance, a wall calendar beside each of our desks, another in the family room, one just inside the garage, the ones on our phones, and a backup one in the guest room.

They are all from 2018 or maybe 2019. Who can remember?

Follow a daily routine. Each evening before going to bed, put the stuff you will always need—your wallet or purse, your keys, phone, glasses, vaccination card, water bottle, newspaper clipping with the Major League Baseball standings from June 1995—in the same place. Each morning try to remember where that place was.

Or better, don't ever leave that place.

Don't forget about it

I'm sure you're wondering what happens if all those strategies don't quite work. What happens if you've tried Post-it notes, mnemonic devices, calendars, mindfulness, and slapping your forehead hard with the palm of your hand—and you still can't remember where your sunglasses are or if you're supposed to take the dog out or if you actually have a dog?

It's probably time then to recognize that your memory may indeed be shot, which happens, but is, of course, a tough pill to swallow, particularly if you are already taking a boatload of vitamin supplements plus that thyroid medication.

In that case, what should you do? How will you cope? Here are a few suggestions that may ameliorate the problems:

If you forget to shut off the water while running a bath, take a shower at the gym instead while your house is being drained.

Can't find your car keys? Always look in the ignition. Can't find the ignition? Please don't drive when I'm on the road.

When you're in the car, and can't remember where you're supposed to be going, pull over to the side of the road, turn on the radio, and listen to a ball game. If it's a baseball game, and it goes into extra innings, and there are a lot of pitching changes, and a number of pinch hitters, by the time it's over you will have remembered where you were going or been arrested. Either way, you'll be able to get home (maybe even with a police escort).

If you keep misplacing your sunglasses, only go out at night, unless you live in the land of the midnight sun, and then you'll just have to recognize you're pretty much screwed.

If you find yourself in the middle of the supermarket and are not sure whether you are supposed to buy fabric softener sheets or sweet Italian sausages, cover your embarrassment by buying both and inventing a new dish.

If you are in that same supermarket aisle and see someone you are sure you absolutely know and just saw yesterday but have no idea who it is, switch to another aisle. I recommend the one with fabric sheets and other cleaning products.

If you are at a cocktail party and are chit-chatting with someone whom you clearly know but just can't come up with that person's name, excuse yourself from the conversation by explaining you need to get another pig-in-a-blanket from the buffet table. If necessary, stuff your mouth with pigs-in-a-blanket if you are asked to introduce that person to someone else whose name you can't remember.

When you can't recollect the name of the actor in that movie whose title you can't recall that also starred the other guy with blonde hair that you may have seen with you-know-who at the beach or maybe it was the mountains, stop watching movies and go read a book instead.

If you can't remember the names of your children or grandchildren, just disinherit all of them and quickly let them know. Their lawyers will remind you of all their names during any depositions.

When you can't recall if you have taken all your pills at breakfast, eat a very early lunch.

Lost track of where you've hidden the good chocolate? Buy more chocolate and hide it pretty much everywhere.

Before you leave the house in the morning, always make sure the kitchen isn't on fire.

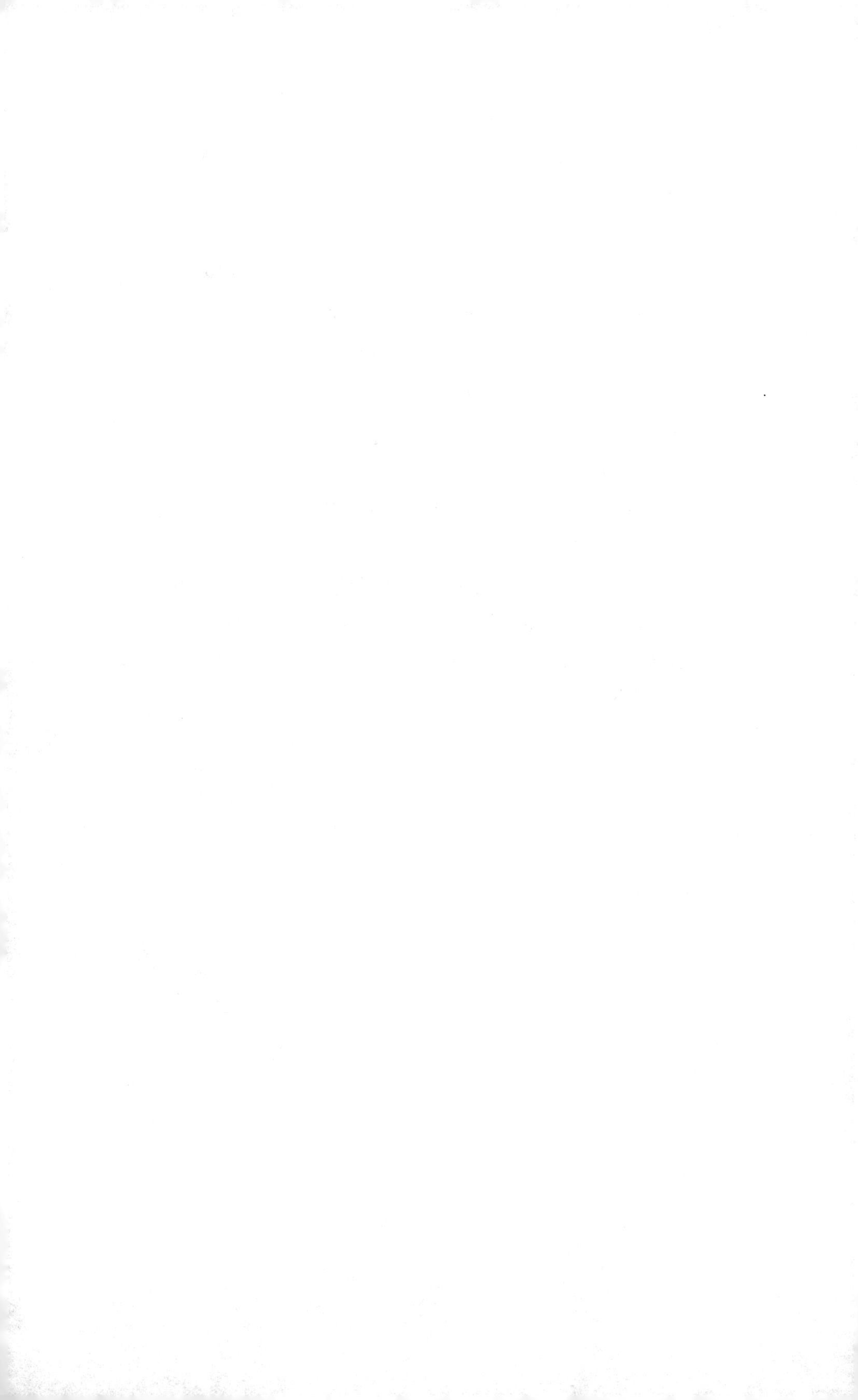

Building a Better Patient

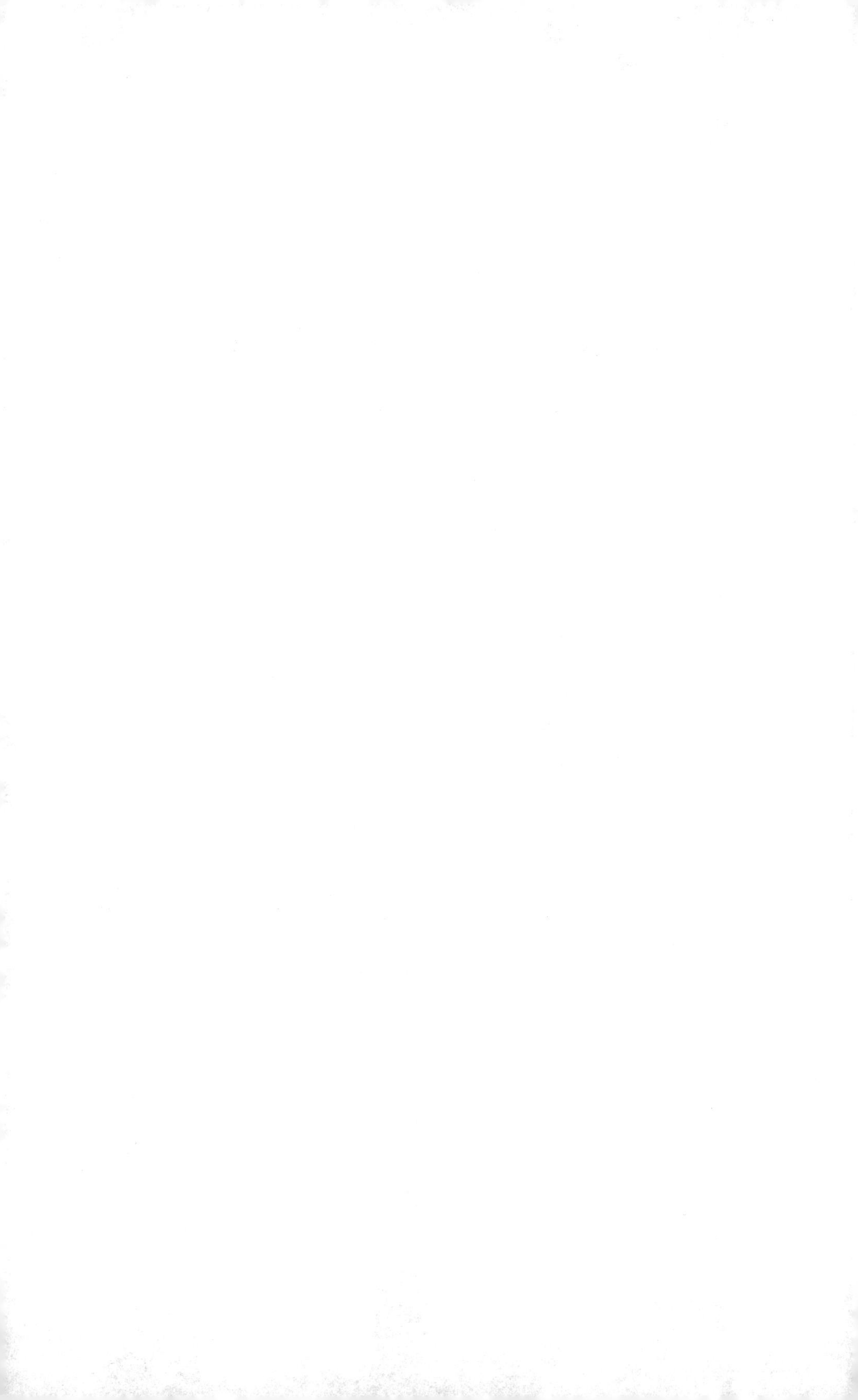

What's up, doc?

Increasingly concerned about the prospect of both physical and mental deterioration, prodded by well-meaning but annoying relatives, and trying to use up our deductible, these days we inevitably wind up in the doctor's office.

Many doctors' offices. Who among us doesn't have a roster something like this?

Dermatologist, podiatrist, cardiologist, urologist, gastroenterologist, orthopedist, therapist, physical therapist, ophthalmologist, radiologist, maybe a nephrologist, and, occasionally, an otolaryngologist which used to be known as an ENT when the co-pay was lower.

And, of course, at the center, our PCP—who used to be known as our GP, when we could get an appointment more easily.

As boomers, we head to our doctors' offices regularly, of

course. Where else can we feel free to complain about a suddenly sore toe and moan about that new ringing in our ears after we have whined so much at home about that excruciating pain in our elbow that family members say they need to go out for some milk and don't return until July?

But getting an appointment with the PCP, or any of the specialists, is not exactly like calling up old Dr. Roginsky (my only doctor until I was twenty or so), and then his coming over to the house a couple of hours later to check out the finger mangled while bowling, a common teenage occupational injury.

Calling for an appointment now might mean having to listen to a robotic voice reminding us to pay careful attention because "our menu options have changed" although they really haven't. Instead, we are encouraged to make all appointments—indeed, have all contact—through the online patient portal. According to the government, which has never had to cancel an 8 a.m. colonoscopy, the portal is "a secure online website that gives patients convenient, 24-hour access to personal health information from anywhere with an Internet connection."

More than 90 percent of medical providers now offer access to a patient portal for their patients, mainly so they never have to talk directly to them. However, only 6 percent of their patients, and only three people beyond the age of fifty-five have any idea at all how the portal works. And 83 percent of boomer patients have been stuck inside their portals for months and can't get out.

As a public service, then, here's how to navigate your portal:

Log in. You will need your name and your password, if you remember your password. If you can't remember your name, call 911. If you enter the password wrong twice before finally getting it right, you will notice on your health summary that your blood pressure is now 173/98.

Go to health summary. You will find this on the home page. The summary is designed to put all your medical information together in one accessible place and to scare the bejeezus out of you when you see your most recent cholesterol numbers and have no idea at all if you should reduce or increase your consumption of omega-3 fatty acids.

Current diagnoses. These generally will be on the right side of the page. They will be listed in formal medicalese so you will be sure you actually have Ebola. The left side will list old diagnoses, so you can feel good that you have successfully navigated puberty.

Medications. Go to the tab at the top that looks like two capsules embracing after a hard day of medicating. All the medications that you have ever taken, even if you stopped taking some of them years ago, will be listed on this page, making you look like some kind of degenerate dope fiend or a Big Pharma bro, which may be the same thing. The medications will be listed with the incomprehensible generic name for your meds so you will have no idea if this particular one is the medicine for your gout or for that time you had werewolf syndrome.

Test results. On this page, you can find the results of all the tests you have taken, such as your bone-density scan, the prostate exam, the colonoscopy, the cholesterol screening, and the PSAT, as long as the tests were administered at this same practice or within the same network. If they were at a different office, practice, or network, you may need a new colonoscopy. Begin the prep soon.

The results of your exams will be written in formulas like 2.3x10E3/uL, so good luck in figuring out what any of it means. After studying the results, you may start to believe that you are suffering from potassium insufficiency or have an overactive epiglottis function, which may or may not be better than an underactive epiglottis function.

Prescriptions. If you want to obtain a new prescription or refill an old one, it makes a lot of sense to go to the page that's called "Prescriptions." It makes no sense to go to the page that's called "Treatments for Werewolf Syndrome" unless you are a preexisting werewolf. At this page, the portal will list the name, address, and contact information for your regular pharmacy. Unfortunately, it's likely to be the wrong name, the wrong address, and the wrong contact information. The good news is that it probably won't be your hair salon.

Messages. This is where you go if you want to send a message to your provider complaining, for instance, that you can't get an appointment within the next six months and that every time you call to talk to your provider you're put on hold and the hold music is instrumental versions of the greatest hits of Strawberry Alarm Clock.

At the messages page, you will be asked if the message is urgent, if it requires a quick reply, or if it is something that they can easily ignore until you start angrily shouting at the portal, which will not answer.

Appointments. After exhausting all the other pages and still not knowing what to do about your chilblains, *finally* click on the tab that will take you to the page where you can try to make an appointment.

The clinic is open on the third Thursday of the month. But, of course, according to the portal, no appointments will be available on any Thursday through the end of the year. There is, however, a slot available on the Thursday that hell freezes over. It's at 6:00 in the morning.

You can keep trying to make an appointment at a better time, on a better day, with a better doctor, but if you're lucky, your portal session time will have already expired.

Side-by-side effects

As we age, we don't just have more doctors' appointments. We gain a number of other things: wisdom, weight, and, of course, prescriptions.

Although many of us prefer now to load up on natural, youthful-seeming supplements—ginger for digestion, turmeric for arthritis, St. John's Wort for worts—we are forced to acknowledge we also probably need more traditional medications, too. That's why sitting on the bathroom counter is that pill that works on our blood pressure, another to balance our thyroid, a third to fix the damage the thyroid pill has done to our blood pressure. And, naturally, the pill that treats the occasional projectile vomiting caused by the combination of all the previous pills.

We need to be extra careful, of course, with all these medications. Particularly after we put on our glasses and read the terrifying warnings buried deep in the information sheets that come with each of the prescriptions.

You may not have noticed, but this is what many of them say:

While taking this medication, unusual dreams may occur, including one where you are dangling naked from a flagpole in the middle of the Roman Forum and being whipped by your first-grade teacher, Miss Bave. If you have had this dream before, decrease your dosage. If you have never had this dream before and would like to, take two extra pills at bedtime.

Get medical help right away if you notice slime coming out of your fingertips or if oatmeal now appears attractive. There could be sudden weight gain, which you will recognize when you can't put on any clothes and you have to go naked to your business meeting at the Roman Forum.

Dizziness and headaches may occur when taking this medication that you are taking for dizziness and headaches. You should not drive, operate heavy machinery, or listen to talk radio while taking this medication until you can do it safely and not scream, "Are you fucking kidding me?"

Discuss with your medical provider immediately any hallucinations you may have about manufacturing a death star while taking your morning medication.

For three days after taking this medication, be careful when you get up from a sitting position and immediately try to drive an M4 Sherman tank. A bout of temporary blindness may follow and if it does, you will not be able to read this list of side effects.

After finishing the required regimen for this drug you are

taking for a condition you didn't know you had until your pinkie got stuck in your nostril, the color of your fingernails should return to normal by Christmas.

Hair loss can occur during the first few months of treatment with this medication. After that, you are likely to grow excessive hair, but mostly on your bedside lamp.

A very serious reaction to this medicine is rare, but that doesn't mean you won't be the one person in 101,886 who actually starts smelling like week-old anchovies.

This medication also may weaken your immune system, making you more susceptible to colds, coughs, COVID-19, and cable-TV reality shows. If you suspect you are watching too much cable-TV reality, call 911 immediately and while waiting for the ambulance to arrive switch to PBS for its thirteen-part series on the history of the cello.

Be sure to drink at least one eight-ounce glass of water with this pill to help minimize the potential loss of the ability to form words.

If you become pregnant while taking this medicine and are a man, reduce activity and contact the *National Enquirer*.

In rare cases, you can die from this medication. It's possible you may prefer that to smelling like week-old anchovies.

And always, remember that your doctor has prescribed this particular medication because he or she is a professional who has scheduled your appointment late in the day and has already seen seventeen other patients who had much more serious issues to deal with, plus lots of insurance paperwork to fill out, and consequently has judged that the benefit to you of this medication is greater than the possibility of projectile vomiting, unless it happens in the waiting room.

This is not a complete list of side effects. If you encounter other side effects not listed above, boy, are you in trouble. If these side effects persist or worsen, contact our lawyers.

In case of emergency

It's possible—even likely—that despite the doctor visits, portal problems, and all the scary medications you take that you may be headed to the emergency room one of these days.

Recent studies have found that those of us older than sixty-five end up in the ER much more often than younger people, who are mostly streaming Apple TV+ or asking ChatGPT to do their taxes. After the age of seventy-five, many of us have established permanent residency in the ER and have started choosing the wallpaper and decorating the bathroom.

Most likely, many of us will wind up in the emergency room in the middle of the night, on a major holiday weekend, when all local medical personnel are attending the annual pickleball injury conference in Hawaii. So, it's important to be prepared for what may be a difficult visit. Here are some suggestions to help get you through it:

Grasp the concept of triage. Triage, from the French for "no matter what you try, you will be waiting for ages," is the preliminary assessment of patients to determine the urgency of their need for treatment. That means, although your ingrown toenail really hurts, you will be seen only after three heart attacks, two gunshot wounds, an epileptic seizure, the kid who swallowed the Silly Putty, and probably the guy with *two* ingrown toenails.

Get your medical story straight. In the ER, you will talk to many different medical personnel. And you will have to repeat the story of who you are and what brings you to the emergency room for all of them, including explaining when you first noticed that your leg had fallen off so they won't want to take another X-ray of your lungs.

Try to understand the lingo. When emergency room personnel tell you your test results will be back soon, make sure you understand that the medical term "soon," when translated into English, really means "not soon." Frequently it means, "not for a very, very long time."

In fact, the whole concept of time is different in the emergency room. New doctors, nurses, and technicians will come and go while you are still there, and then they will come back again after having gone home for the holidays, headed off to Cancun, and renewed their driver's licenses.

Don't be wearing your pajamas when you have to go to the emergency room. For one thing, what are you doing in pajamas at two in the afternoon while taking a walk around the neighborhood? Once in the emergency room, the likelihood is that if you arrive in your pajamas, you will stay in your pajamas. And you will have to do a lot of explaining why a person your age still has Lady and the Tramp pajamas.

Bring a board game with you. You need something to kill the time and take your mind off the blood that's been trickling down your leg and the throbbing in your chest. Consider Scrabble, and try to get "triage" on a triple-word space.

Respond honestly to the questions you are asked. While you are flat on your back on a gurney with multiple tubes coming out of your arm, a bandage wrapped around your elbow, and a thumping in your chest, do not respond, "fine, thanks, and you?" when medical personnel introduce themselves by saying, "How are you?"

Don't believe that it's all some sort of terrible mistake. Acknowledge that you are in the ER for a reason. Yes, you work out regularly, do yoga twice a week, kick-boxing every other Thursday, haven't smoked since college, and can regularly complete *The New York Times* crossword—*in pen.* But you are, after all, old enough to distinctly remember where you were when JFK was shot.

Keep things in perspective. Do not be concerned that most of the medical practitioners you are seeing at the ER are the same age as many of your t-shirts. Be nice to them. They probably *have* gone to medical or nursing school, and even if they can't help you with whatever problem has brought you to the ER, you might have played poker with their grandparents.

Caring about Medicare

As we age, just as important as our health but with more forms to fill out is our health insurance. Whether at the doctor's office or the emergency room, we need health insurance, and choosing the correct kind is a complicated process requiring a deep understanding of how we are likely to be fleeced at any moment.

If you're not yet sixty-five, you probably have private or employer health insurance and have not bothered to read the fine print on your insurance card while you still can see the fine print without squinting. Basically, the fine print says that your best insurance plan is to plan not to get sick.

Meanwhile, your premium has been going up and your employer's contribution has been going down, so many of us look forward to the day we finally can be covered by Medicare. For boomers, being able to enroll in Medicare is one of the major benefits of getting older, right after qualifying for the senior discount at the supermarket.

Like many of us, I thought enrolling in Medicare would be easy. I figured I'd have to prove I was sixty-five by remembering who won Super Bowl III (the New York Jets) and who was the Beatles' drummer before Ringo Starr (Pete Best), but then I'd automatically be covered because that was the American way.

Well, not exactly. Just like the American way, with its tolls every few miles, dangerous curves up ahead, and lack of a single clean rest stop, Medicare has co-pays every few visits, dangerous deductibles up ahead, and also not a single clean rest stop.

Let me explain, for those of you already enrolled and hopelessly confused and for those of you who are younger and looking forward to becoming hopelessly confused.

Medicare is actually not one whole plan but many different parts. The first part is Part A and sometimes Part B. Then there's the party of the second part, which is Part C and Part D. Altogether, sort of, these parts are colloquially called "Original Medicare." Because, why not?

Medicare Part A is essentially hospital insurance. You insure the hospital you won't need to go there often. If you appear too frequently, you pay full price for one surgery but at least get the second one 50 percent off.

Medicare Part B covers certain doctors' services but only ones you will probably never need. These include what is generally known as outpatient care, which means you generally will be out a good bit of money.

Medicare Part A doesn't cost anything, which is probably why it doesn't cover much of anything. You actually do pay for Part B, with your premium set each year by a group of actuaries bored with playing fantasy football.

Then there's Medicare Part C. Well, technically, there is no Medicare Part C.

It's just called Part C, sometimes, to further mystify us in case we weren't already so mystified we have started eating our soup with a fork. Part C is more commonly called a Medicare Advantage Plan. Advantage plans are offered by a private insurer that has made a sweetheart deal with Medicare, which was too busy writing confusing enrollment guidelines to pay attention.

Designed to make up the difference between what Medicare pays and what the federal deficit is, an Advantage plan provides all the Part A and Part B benefits, plus, maybe, a side of fries. Most also provide Medicare Part D benefits, which is prescription drug coverage because it would have been too simple to call it Medicare prescription drug benefits.

There's also a Dual Complete Plan, which is like an Advantage plan but may be something entirely different after all is said and done or it could be the exact same thing under a different name because health insurance companies want to keep us on our toes. These plans cover 20 percent of this and 35 percent of that or 100 percent of something else (after the first 35 percent) and 60 percent of the second 25 percent, minus the 18 percent co-pay, for days one to six if you are an inpatient and can read the third line of the eye chart. Assuming, of course, you are in network.

Then there's a Medicare Supplement Plan, which is different from a Medicare Advantage Plan because it does not include Plan D prescription coverage but does include everything else and doesn't make you pay co-pays after you meet your deductible, which you could do some enchanted evening across a crowded room. A Medicare Supplement Plan is also sometimes called a Medigap Plan in a largely successful effort to give many of us migraine headaches.

If you get a supplement plan, you will have to get a separate Part D prescription plan, but there may be none left because you have taken so much time figuring out all the previous parts.

Many different private insurance companies offer these supplement plans. Each company tells you its supplement plan is better than every other insurance company's supplement plan. In fact, they are all exactly the same because the government requires them to be exactly the same but the companies don't want to tell you that because it might actually help you make a decision instead of slapping yourself upside the head trying to choose among them.

If you are confused by all this, and also don't understand how which plan you can get and how much you will pay for it also will depend on where you live, how old you are, if you ever smoked or attended a KISS concert, and whether you are still breathing, be comforted by the fact that you have made the insurance companies very happy.

By the way, you can only enroll in any of these plans during a precise period of the year, called the open enrollment period. If you try to enroll outside that time, you will be made to pay a higher premium and forced to read the 723-page Medicare Annual Notice of Changes in its entirety.

Choose your coverage

Even within Medicare, there are choices to be made. To help you decide in which health insurance plan to actually enroll, let us review our coverage options.

You can choose a health maintenance organization (an HMO), a preferred provider organization (a PPO) or a direct underwritten medical brotherhood organization (a DUMBO).

There's also a D-SNP plan (absolutely no idea what that stands for), which could be an HMO plan, although it's possible it could also be a PPO plan. And there are, as we all know, five types of D-SNPs: All-Dual, Full-Benefit, Medicare Zero Cost-Sharing, Dual Eligible Subset, and Dual Eligible Subset Medicare Zero Cost-Sharing. (At the end of the open-enrollment period, there's a test and you will have to repeat all the variations, in order. Winners receive a Visa card for zero cost-sharing of any debilitating illness of their choice.)

Once you decide on your overall plan, you will need to determine which tier of the plan to choose.

Your insurer's Pewter Plan offers a smaller deductible and larger co-pay, depending on whether you want to see just a regular doctor or a specialist who will want to know if you've ever had a fungal infection and what was so special about it.

The Brass Plan covers more services but requires a higher out-of-pocket cost and a more restrictive limit on how much you will pay for those covered services, which are services that take place under a cover, such as an umbrella.

The Silver Plan has lower co-pays but higher co-insurance and no one in customer service who is able to lucidly explain the difference between the two.

Then there's the Gold Plan, which has no deductible, no co-pays, no co-insurance, but requires that you pay in gold.

Under these plans, the cost of services will change if you are in network, out of network, or prefer One America News Network because you are convinced Medicare is a deep state conspiracy.

If you are out of sorts but in network, there will be an annual medical deductible that will begin only after you have exhausted all your patience and some other patients. There will be a separate deductible for your medications, just because they can.

Reimbursement for your medications will work like this:

If your drugs fall into the Tier 1 grouping, the cost will be minimal because you are really getting only a placebo and all employees of the pharmacy have been sworn to secrecy about it.

If your drugs fall into Tier 2, which are generally generic medications, the cost will be more or less generic as these medications may help you somewhat more than feeding a cold and/or starving a fever would. Or they may not.

If your drugs fall into Tier 3, you will pay 12 percent of the actual cash price of the medication, which is the price you paid for your house. That means the medications should be taken with food but you are forbidden to refinance while chewing.

If your drugs fall into Tier 4, you will pay what is called the full Rx price, which is 23 percent of the research and development cost of the drug, multiplied by the LIBOR, or London Interbank Offered Rate, on the first day of the preceding month. Also, you may have to explain to the pharmacist why you have not been put into immediate quarantine.

If your drugs fall into Tier 5, don't worry about paying for the drugs. You have more important things to worry about.

Building a Better Build

The shape of things

Exercise more. Sleep better. Improve our diet.

Yeah, yeah, yeah. Nag, nag, nag. This is the kind of advice we keep hearing, again and again, from doctors and magazine articles and TV commercials and doctors who write magazine articles and appear in TV commercials. But the fact is, we *know* all this already. We know what we are supposed to do to stay as youthful as possible, as sharp as necessary, and extend our lifespans, or at least remain somewhat fit and sentient until there's a new season of *Succession*.

Why else would so many of us play pickleball? Or eat vegan pickles?

We know that with the potential physical and cognitive decline that can come with aging, exercise, in particular, has become crucial. Living longer and living better means we really should exercise even if it kills us.

By working out for just a few minutes a day, we are told,

we can become fit enough so we're not out of breath each time we open the mail. We can improve muscle tone to the point where we are not too embarrassed to go to the beach in the summer or the gym in the winter or the botanical gardens in the spring, unless the allergies start acting up again and we're out of tissues.

Exercise can help us lose the weight we have spent forty years carefully accumulating, tone those abs, and streamline those glutes, assuming the glutes are where we think they are. Vigorous physical activity, in fact, ultimately can keep our bodies the finely tuned machines they never really were but we'd like to imagine they once might have been.

Plus, exercise not just tones the body, as a bonus it also engages the brain, and thus can take your mind off how annoyed you feel actually having to exercise. Instead of worrying about that lingering pain in the lower back, exercise can help you focus instead on any new troublesome throbbing in your chest when you try to do the plank.

Exercise can stimulate endorphins, those neurotransmitters that interact with receptors in the brain to reduce the perception of pain, so you don't notice how painful exercise is. [Nevertheless, be forewarned: No matter how many endorphins you're releasing, you still will find Netflix's *Emily in Paris* painful.]

All those new neurons firing in the brain might finally account for that headache you've had since 2013 and that odd smoky smell every time you try to concentrate and figure out your share of an 18 percent tip at a takeout-only restaurant.

Moreover, exercise lowers the risk of high blood pressure

and diabetes and can help us sleep better, as long as we don't try to nap while on the treadmill, and can help with balance issues, as long as we don't try to do pushups while on the elliptical.

In general, vigorous physical activity actually slows the aging process and just makes you feel better, more youthful, and greatly superior to anyone who's still stuck on the couch watching old *Jeopardy* reruns because they were unnaturally fond of Alex Trebek.

So, forget those battered knees and that plantar fasciitis and get out there now and lift a Subaru! Who cares if you can't stay awake between lunch and dinner—go run a marathon! Take up kick-boxing! Do squats with a kettle ball while swimming laps during a Zumba class! Beat up your neighbor! It'll get your target heart rate up, particularly when the police arrive.

And remember that for every minute of exercise we do during our lifetime, there will be one less minute to dread exercising, which is clearly a win-win.

Exercising our demons

But what kind of exercise? According to a new study published in either *The Journal of the American Medical Association* or *Teen People*, aging patients who met the guidelines of at least thirty minutes of moderate exercise five times a week found that they did not have to make believe they actually like kale to appear younger and healthier.

Okay, but what exactly is moderate exercise?

Lifting light-to-medium weights, such as the plate you're carrying back from the endless salad bar. Repetitive squatting, when you've dropped your glasses and can't find them because you're not wearing your glasses. Or walking, for instance.

Walking is a simple exercise that almost anyone can learn to do if they have two feet and know how to alternate them. I personally prefer left-right-left, but I understand there are some who support right-left-right, even though they are wrong. In the spirit of bipartisanship, we are willing to let it go.

You can walk almost any time of the day, during any season, and at any longitude, except 37.5412 degrees, which is in the middle of the Atlantic Ocean. Walking reduces blood pressure, lowers cholesterol, and gets you out of the house when there is cleaning to be done. It also can get your target heart rate up.

(If you have no idea what your target heart rate is and how to find it, take your resting heart rate—the rate you have when barely listening to your lawyer explain the provisions of your will and suggesting you buy long-term care insurance—and multiply that by the number of medications you take on a regular basis, not including vitamins or other supplements, and then subtract how many times you want to nap before it's even noon. Remember to always exercise at about 85 percent of your target heart rate or 73 percent more than you'd prefer to be doing.)

Walkers should aim for taking 10,000 steps a day. To break that down into specifics, it means that every minute of the day you must take at least 6.95 steps, even if you are sleeping, eating, or reading studies published in *Teen People*. Taking 10,000 steps each day typically burns about 2,000 to 3,500 extra calories each week or about 13,500 extra calories per month (except in February) or about 156,000 extra calories per year, which equates to four servings of Breyers Mint Chocolate Chip ice cream.

If you want six servings, consider sleepwalking.

If you have missed a day and taken no steps, because

you've been lying in bed since early in the morning scrolling through Facebook and getting annoyed that other people are taking cruises around the Greek islands, remember that you can always do catch-up contributions by running for hours around the bed.

How to get started

It can be difficult to get started on an exercise regimen, particularly if we prefer sitting on the couch and reading obituaries and noticing with alarm how many obituary subjects are younger than we are. So here then are a few common-sense suggestions on how to help launch a new fitness plan and fit all this essential physical activity into an already busy day of eating and napping.

First, assess your fitness level. And don't be too discouraged if you find out you have no fitness level. At least you still have blood pressure. Got a pulse, right? Can still remember the plot of the last episode of *Game of Thrones*? You're good.

Consider your fitness goals. Do you want to be able to walk to the mailbox without getting out of breath? Swim the Pacific? Leap tall buildings in a single bound? At first, it's always best to try for something attainable but just a little bit beyond your current grasp. Consider your neighbor's mailbox.

Plan to include different activities. This is also known as cross-training and has dual benefits. It can keep you from getting bored with whatever exercise you have chosen and can reduce your chances of injuring or overusing one specific muscle or joint. This way, you can injure and overuse all your muscles and joints at the same time, saving you separate co-pays at the ER.

Put it on paper. Write down your goals. A written plan may encourage you to stay on track. It also may encourage you to go get a bag of pretzels and watch Wolf Blitzer announce "breaking news!" instead.

Start slow and progress slowly. You don't have to run a marathon that first week you start exercising. Instead, walk out to the mailbox. If you feel you're hitting the wall, you may have gone the wrong way.

Build exercise activity into your daily routine. When you wake up in the middle of the night, be sure to run to the bathroom. Button your shirts with ten-pound weights attached to your pinkies. Do twenty-five squats any morning you intend to pay your utility bills.

Turn your commute into a workout. If you are driving, whenever you come to a red light, get out of the car, run around your vehicle twice, and then if the traffic has moved on, get into someone else's car and ask them to drop you at the office. This also has social benefits and keeps you engaged with the community.

Exercise at work. Instead of sitting immobile staring

at a monitor, every fifteen minutes or so get up and start swinging a kettlebell around. This works best, of course, when you are working at home, in your bedroom, and your supervisor and colleagues are not standing right next to you. (If you happen to be at the office, always remember to apologize to any concussed coworkers you have kettlebelled.)

Sneak in a workout during your lunch break. Order a very large pastrami on rye sandwich. Lift it over your head five times. Rest. Lift the pickle.

Allow time for recovery. There's a rule of thumb for this: if your thumb hurts after exercise, take it easy and go have a beer. Use the other thumb to lift it.

Find a fitness buddy. I recommend my friend Rob, who hates exercise as much as I do and also would prefer getting a beer and a couple of donuts.

And remember—before you start any exercise program, check with your medical providers. If you're lucky, maybe they will stop you.

Witness to fitness

In a discussion the other day at the gym with my personal trainer, I asked one very obvious question: What am I doing with a personal trainer? What are any of us doing with a personal trainer?

Acting on the advice of our medical providers, many boomers have joined gyms—also known as fitness centers if the monthly payment is more than your mortgage—because we finally get it: it's exercise that will keep us healthy, extend our lifespans, and perhaps help us identify a song by Megan Thee Stallion.

Gyms help us get stronger, particularly in our core. As we grow older, we need to focus on improving our core strength because strong core muscles keep us balanced and stable, making it easier to perform many of our favorite activities, such as arguing with the cable company. They help us bend down to tie our shoes and get up from seated positions after six hours of bingeing The Weather Channel. They prevent lower-back problems and keep our minds focused on upper digestive system reflux. Most important, they help fight off the awareness of ongoing physical and mental deterioration, mainly because when your core hurts, you can't concentrate on anything else.

Many of us also join gyms for the sense of camaraderie. We like being among others who are focused on improving their bodies and also can't do two chin-ups. A few of us join gyms because some have saunas or steam rooms and we like to sit in there watching other baby boomers schvitz, which is the Yiddish word for sweating while complaining about how your core hurts.

Others go to the gym for the fitness classes, where you can listen to earsplitting music while pretending you're almost replicating the moves of the younger people in the front row.

I joined a gym through a program for seniors called Silver Sneakers, named after our hair color and a much better name than Bald Sneakers. It's a program designed to get older people more active, and, in the words of its website, "defy the odds, shatter stereotypes and answer every challenge with, 'I can do this!'"

Like a lot of boomers, I was pretty sure I couldn't do this, but, hey, Silver Sneakers was free—except for the $325 monthly health insurance premium I had to pay to get the free perk—so I joined a local gym.

But gyms, as many of us have noticed, can be intimidating places full of younger people with bulging muscles and muscular tattoos. Don't be afraid. Remember, you once used to look like that, except for the tattoos and the muscles part.

The gyms are also filled with exercise machines that may appear to have been directly imported from the Spanish Inquisition. While those muscular younger people were in the corner of the gym lifting Subaru Outbacks over their heads, I found myself a personal trainer because, not surprisingly, I needed someone to explain how to not hurt myself while lifting my own Outback.

(Of course, like many of us, I also liked saying I had a personal trainer, which sounds so much better than referring to "my dental hygienist" or "my atrial fib tech.")

My personal trainer, obviously, was trim, muscular and younger than most of my t-shirts. She first made sure I was in excellent shape for a 106-year-old nearsighted lifetime smoker with fallen arches. She tested my current fitness level by having me run on a treadmill, squat in place, do as many pushups as I could in one minute and then see if I could remember my name.

While I was alternating between gasping for breath and wheezing for breath, she went through a description of all the complicated machines out there on the gym floor, not including the vending machine, which I already knew how to operate. She explained carefully how to set them all up and outlined the right technique, which muscle groups each of them worked and what emergency number to call when I got my finger stuck between the weights.

Each machine, she explained, was specially designed to strengthen you, firm you up, and make you regret not having done any pushups since seventh grade. Each machine targeted a particular area of the body that somehow you may not already have abused by accident.

Maybe you've had this experience: After the personal trainer left to explain to another Silver Sneakers member how to press the button and turn on an elliptical machine, I remembered nothing much about how the exercise machines actually worked.

Should your elbows be level with the pivot points or your hands be just above the shoulder grips, but only when you are crying out in pain? Should you sit up straight with head back against the top pad or should you crunch over with heels together and knees bent so you could hurt more than one muscle at a time?

When I left the gym, my confusion was total, but my Subaru Outback was waiting outside. Instead of lifting it, however, I had barely enough strength left to put it in drive.

Work those quads!

Yes, the gym can be a scary place, particularly for those of us whose idea of exercise is manually switching from Hulu to HBO Max and who are also too embarrassed to ask what glutes are exactly. It really doesn't have to be that way, as long as you understand how these machines work, exactly what you're supposed to do with them, and what grievous injuries they can cause.

Here's some help.

Bicep Curl

Adjust the seat to the appropriate height and make your weight selection. That's the weight you want to curl, not the weight you plan to weigh after finally eliminating Oreos from your diet.

Place your upper arms against the pads and grasp the handles. This will be your starting position. It's also likely to be the ending position because you probably won't be able to move your arms.

Perform the movement, if you can, by flexing the elbow, pulling your lower arm toward your upper arm. Hold that position. Scream in pain.

Pec Fly

Adjust the seat so the handles are slightly below your elbows but above your knees and close to your kidneys (right above your spleen, wherever that is). Rotate the hand grips until you can't feel your fingers. As you make coordinated movements until the pain in your neck is excruciating, try to figure out what a pec is and how you could make it fly.

Chest Extension/Leg Curl

Choose your weight and sit on the machine with your legs under the pad (feet pointed forward, teeth clenched, brain hyperventilating) and hands holding the side bars with mouth rounded to better allow you to shout for help. This will be your starting position.

If the angle of your elbow is less than ninety degrees, that means your ulna is already dislocated and you should go to the emergency room as soon as possible, or after you do ten reps, whichever comes first.

Triceps Extension/Seated Dip/Abdominal Crunch

Make sure you adjust the knee pad of the machine to fit

your height and prevent you from flying across the gym floor and into the sauna before you've requested a towel.

Have both arms extended in front of you, holding the bar at the chosen grip width, then bring your torso back around thirty degrees until you hear something crack. Exhale loudly, so staff will come quickly with the stretcher.

Hip Abductor/Hip Adductor/Triceps Press

The upper torso should remain stationary, the lower torso should be frozen in fear, and only the arms should move while you whimper.

Lateral Raise/Seated Chest Contortioner

Breathe out when you bring the bar down until it touches your upper chest before shouting for help. Work your pecs, your delts, and your glutes. If you do not know your delts from your glutes, be careful while putting on your pants.

Shoulder Hoist/Leg Press/Triceps Twirl

Adjust the pad so that it falls on top of your lower leg (just above the scar from the hip abductor/hip adductor/triceps press). Also, make sure your legs form a ninety-degree angle so you can get up from the machine quickly before it comes crashing down.

Lat Press

Press your lats close to the point where you can feel the tension between your desire to be home reading a trashy murder mystery on your Kindle and your embarrassment that other people in the gym might be watching you.

Pause at the top of the movement, and then slowly return the weight to the starting position. Take a deep breath, slowly exhale, and then cancel your gym membership.

Run for your life

UNFORTUNATELY, MODERATE EXERCISE MAY NOT BE enough if we really want to become truly fit and guarantee that we'll be around for the launch of the iPhone 93 Pro. In addition to moderate exercise, we have been advised many, many times that we should aim for at least thirty minutes of high-intensity aerobic activity four or five days a week.

(This advice comes from medical providers, spouses who have read too many health blogs, and "wellness coaches," which is a new profession that combines psychology, counseling, and high-energy nagging.)

Aerobic exercise is technically exercise that requires pumping of oxygenated blood by the heart to deliver oxygen to working muscles. Aerobic exercises, for example, would be jogging, swimming, sled dog mushing—particularly if you're the dog—or screaming at the television set during a presidential press conference. In other words, it's exercise that makes your heart and lungs really work and make you gasp for breath and unable to finish a sent . . .

Although there are many different kinds of aerobic exercise, what they all have in common is that you will probably dislike them at first. Probably at second, too. Nevertheless, you will likely end up overdoing it because overdoing is what we do. In desperate attempts to keep up, look good, and, preferably, not die, we boomers frequently undertake extreme physical challenges even though we are somewhat aware that the challenges are, technically, completely nuts.

Very much in this spirit, I decided not long ago I was going to run a half marathon. (Many of us have even considered the idea of running full marathons, until younger and smarter people helpfully have pointed out to us "that's 26.2 miles, *moron.*" It's also 42.16 kilometers or, in England, 16.7 imperial liters.)

A half marathon, it seemed to me, would be slightly more achievable and, I convinced myself, would really improve my aerobic fitness, unleash a boatload of endorphins, lower my blood pressure, slim my body, sharpen my brain, and prove that I am still every bit as dumb as I was when I thought that smoking a pipe at the age of eighteen obscured my acne and made me look more mature.

Like many of us of a certain age, I wanted to test my mettle and find out if, in fact, I had any mettle left and if that was the reason I was having so much difficulty getting through security control at airports.

Some of us have chosen to challenge ourselves in other ways—competing in triathlons, hiking the Inca Trail, mowing the lawn without sunscreen, or opening email attachments from unknown sources.

For my new challenge, I had considered ice swimming and calf roping, and calf roping while ice swimming, but ultimately chose to run the half marathon. What a thrill it would be to run so far and demonstrate to everyone that age is just a number, although younger people may think it's a noun.

Running a half marathon, I knew, would require stamina, fortitude, and a high tolerance for pain. On the other hand, it would offer the opportunity to buy expensive new exercise gear, which remains one of the main reasons most of us boomers exercise.

I opted first for running shoes with the antipronating roll bar, the loft cushioning, the DNA midsole, the soft leather uppers, and the air mesh inner soles because, naturally, that was the first pair the store clerk showed me and I didn't want to embarrass myself in front of an eighteen-year-old who didn't even smoke a pipe. I also purchased the obligatory coordinated headbands, wristbands, calf sleeves, and reflector patches.

Now fully equipped, I decided to run for practice a popular 5K race before the half marathon. I chose this particular 5K because it attracted several hundred competitors, increasing my chances of not finishing dead last or worse, last and dead.

I found my place at the back of the racers, right next to a guy wearing full chain mail, a type of armor. He also carried a lance and was wearing heavy boots. That was, I had to acknowledge, even better than calf sleeves and reflector patches.

I didn't care if he was completely nuts because I thought I might actually beat him to the finish. Assuming he'd be slow and plodding, I figured I could put on a (relative) burst of speed near the end and shoot ahead.

The starting gun went off. My wife, there to cheer me on and to remind me to be careful and don't do too much and for God's sake, be careful, waved excitedly at me. I stopped to wave back, immediately falling behind every single other runner, some of whom had already finished the race.

As we rounded the final turn toward the finish line, I accelerated: a poetic metaphor for not going quite as slowly as I had before. As a result, I was able to cross the finish line seconds ahead of the guy in armor.

Exulting in my triumph, I shouted out, "I'm number 764!" Then the guy in armor whom I had beaten was greeted at the finish line by, honest, another guy in armor who had already finished long ago and was casually eating an orange.

Later, I did find out that I had finished second in my age group. Of course, there were only two of us in our age group. Everybody else was dead or at home watching the Golf Channel.

Last lap

I HAVE TO CONFESS: I NEVER DID RUN THAT HALF marathon.

This frequently happens to boomers. We start off with the best of intentions and then remember we have Netflix and there may be some Italian sorbetto in the freezer. We want to keep up, get back in shape, show everybody how youthful we still are, and stave off impending decrepitude, but then we find out there are crossword puzzles we haven't finished yet and naps that need to be taken.

Plus, who has time to train when you can find clips of the old Sunday night *Ed Sullivan Show* somewhere on the internet? Half marathon or hating on Topo Gigio? Practice run or rolling your eyes at Totie Fields?

It's a very easy call.

Does this trajectory sound familiar? I had bought a GPS-enabled watch to track my runs and mock me for not knowing what my VO2 max was. I had purchased special sweat-absorbing socks that came with their own sweat. I had almost gotten pierced by a lance and humiliated by a crusades reenactor with too much time on his chain-mailed hands. And yet despite it all, I still had difficulty correctly spelling plantar fasciitis.

I decided I had had enough.

Wanting to run the half marathon was the kind of physical challenge we accept in an attempt to stay younger and it probably would be, I thought, less messy than dyeing my hair green. It would help my cardiovascular functioning and would be simpler than trying to figure out my Body Mass Index number. Despite my age, despite an increasingly large bald spot, it would show my youthful determination, my boyish perseverance and, of course, my utter cluelessness.

But I never did run it, and there's a lesson to be learned here for all of us. Trying to remain young or at least trying to seem young is hard work. It's much easier if you already are young. Running a half marathon would mean, I finally realized, *running* a half marathon, which is a lot more difficult than a leisurely stroll to the mailbox.

Like many boomers trying to recapture our youth, my reach had exceeded my grasp a bit too much, which meant I really hurt my shoulder while reaching and needed several months of PT and lessons in alternative grasping.

Because we are at a point in our lives when we feel we have more free time and are no longer encumbered by demanding jobs or growing families or accumulating small kitchen appliances that we'll never use, we foolishly think we have the opportunity to do what we may always have wanted to do: run a (half) marathon, hike Everest, write that novel, or learn Python (yeah, I don't know what it is either).

Instead, let's understand that we have probably missed that boat—even if we have seriously considered the Danube River cruise package— and need to be more realistic about our goals. We need instead to focus on potentially more attainable objectives, like maybe sleeping through the night.

Building a Better Sleeper

Losing our snoozing

We all know it, we should get enough sleep. But as we get older we sleep less and frequently sleep badly—and that affects...well, pretty much everything.

Chronic sleep deprivation can lead to high blood pressure, diabetes, dementia, and staying awake at night worrying about chronic sleep deprivation. Lack of adequate sleep can contribute to increased risk of heart disease and serial yawning during presentations on exchange traded funds by your financial advisor.

Sleep deprivation hinders the body's immune responses and thwarts the brain's ability to organize memories, which is why you can't remember where you put some of those memories. It ages the skin and puts wrinkles on our wrinkles. It can lead to poor judgment, like accepting spam calls about an expired car warranty from somebody in Billings, MT, or purchasing a high-fee, low-return annuity from that financial advisor, even during a bear market.

It can even cause weight gain. When you're sleep deprived, your body increases the hormone that tells you you're hungry while decreasing the hormone that controls your appetite. Also, since you're sleeping less, you have more time to snack on Little Debbie's.

Most of all, not getting enough sleep makes us tired.

And it dominates our conversations.

When we get up in the morning, much too early in the morning, we talk about how we couldn't sleep during the night.

My wife, for instance, notes that she awoke at 1:45 a.m., 3:19, and for good at 6:53. Competitive as always, I counter with taking 43 minutes to fall asleep, waking up at 2:57, and then waking for good—or rather for worse—at 5:19. I am the winner, or rather the loser.

We aren't forced to get up early anymore because most of us don't have to commute to work or get the kids off to school. We're getting up early because we're tired of lying in bed counting sheep or medical conditions we need to mention to our doctors.

According to a report from the Johns Hopkins School of Daily Dozing, not sleeping well is a classic sign of aging, right up there with needing to go to the bathroom right after you've gone to the bathroom. Aging boomers definitely have a much harder time falling asleep and even more trouble staying asleep than when we were younger. In our twenties and thirties, we could sleep until noon, at least partially because we didn't go to bed until three in the morning. Sometimes we could sleep until February because, after all, it was the sixties (or it's possible we weren't actually sleeping but totally zonked out of our minds).

Now, many of us haven't been sleeping well for years. We don't get enough rest because we have so much on our minds —global climate change, the rise of fascism, the immigration crisis, that worrisome new fluttering in our chest, and whether we turned off the oven. Mostly, we're worried that when we go to bed we may not wake up. And then, of course, once we finally do get to sleep, we frequently have to get up in the middle of the night to go pee, trying to do it in the dark, and occasionally missing the target.

Also, technically speaking, as we age the master clock in a part of the brain called the hypothalamus, known more informally as the suprachiasmatic nucleus, regulates our sleep cycles, or circadian rhythms. As the nucleus gets creaky and has difficulty concentrating on the paragraph it's reading, our circadian rhythms get out of whack.

If we're unable to find any whack, which happens when you get older because you can't find where you've put anything, our bodies begin to produce lower levels of growth hormone, so we are likely to experience a decrease in slow wave or deep sleep, which is an especially refreshing part of the sleep cycle and was voted No. 1 sleep cycle in an AARP survey. When this happens we produce less melatonin, meaning we'll often experience more fragmented sleep and wake up more often during the night because we need to drive to the 24-hour Walgreens to pick up a case of melatonin.

These problems can be exacerbated by certain medicines we now take, which are designed to counter the side effects of other medicines we now take. Or maybe it's that we just have to go to the bathroom a lot more or have run out of sheep to count and start wondering, while we're lying restlessly in bed, do sheep who can't sleep count people?

Dreaming of dozing

WHATEVER THE CAUSES OF BAD OR INSUFFICIENT SLEEP, it's vital to improve our sleep hygiene if we want to live longer and better or at least not fall asleep while we're taking a shower or running that 5K.

What is good sleep hygiene? Hint: it doesn't mean washing your hands and face and brushing your teeth before you go to sleep, although it really wouldn't hurt, you know? Consider cleaning your nails, too.

Actually, according to the National Snoring Foundation, good sleep hygiene is a variety of different practices and habits that are necessary to have good nighttime sleep quality and full daytime alertness. It means preparing for sleep in an organized manner and giving yourself the best possible situation to allow you to fall asleep and stay asleep until it is time to take your nap.

Every lifestyle magazine, every digital newsletter, and every AARP bulletin tells us we must follow the rules of good sleep hygiene if we want to sleep better and sleep longer and thus live better and live longer and be able to watch our grandchildren grow up and ignore us. Reading all these recommendations can be terribly boring, although reading them actually might put you to sleep.

But with naps to take and medications to swallow, who has time for all that reading? So, I've boiled them down for you. Here then are the top seventeen sleep hygiene rules we have to follow:

Develop a sleep routine. Do anything that relaxes you before heading to bed: take a warm shower, spend a few moments meditating, or quietly pop open a bag of Doritos. Create a bedtime ritual, doing the same things in the same order so you are telling your brain and your body that it's time to wind down. For some, this might include taking a warm bath, then listening to soothing music while launching a drone attack.

Stick to that same sleep schedule. For instance, go to bed at the same time every night, unless that means falling asleep just when you are driving home and coming down the ramp onto the interstate. In that case, if you do fall asleep, stay in the right lane after merging.

Plan also on getting up at the same time every morning, preferably in the same place. When the switch to daylight savings time comes around, just acknowledge that you are screwed.

Create a sleep sanctuary. Make sure your bedroom environment is soothing and comfortable and is not on the parade route of a marching band. Your bedroom should be a haven of comfort, which means removing all the dirty dishes from under your pillows. You want to create a room that is dark, quiet, comfortable, and preferably has a bed in it.

Eat lightly in the evening. You don't want your digestive system working hard while you are trying to power down. Heavy or rich foods, fatty or fried meals, spicy dishes, citrus fruits, carbonated drinks, and all the other stuff we really like can trigger indigestion, which can interfere with sleep. On the other hand, sleep can also interfere with enjoying spicy dishes and fried foods, so this will really be a tough call.

Don't drink alcoholic beverages late at night. They can interfere with your sleep, so better start your drinking early in the day.

Watch your caffeine intake. Caffeine can remain in your system longer than you might realize. That cup you drank during sophomore year in college? Still there. That espresso you had while on vacation in Italy, so you could impress the waiter who had just laughed at your Italian accent? Yup, still there, and still making fun of your accent.

Don't take naps. You will enjoy them too much and think about them all the time while you can't sleep.

Before going to bed, stay away from electronic devices. Don't stare at that smartphone, tablet, or computer screen, unless there's a really interesting Twitter/X thread or something on Facebook about how to buy the best electric can openers.

Be wary of watching TV as part of your bedtime ritual. Some research suggests that watching TV before bedtime interferes with sleep, particularly if it is Fox News or reruns of *The Walking Dead*, which may be the same thing.

Avoid bright lights before bed, particularly those of a police interrogation room.

Do not eat Mallomar cookies in bed. There are, however, exceptions to this rule, like Wednesdays and Sundays.

Do not Zoom after 10 p.m. Especially do not do this with people who can't figure out how to mute themselves.

Don't text anyone late at night. They will probably text you back and you will have to text them back and this could go on all night and you'll never get to bed though at least you will have the last word.

Never go to sleep angry. Stay up and fight. Shout threateningly at the phone when the Delta Airlines customer service digital voice tells you their agents are currently helping other customers and the current wait time is eight and a half hours. Argue with people on Twitter/X who have only three followers but sincerely believe they understand macroeconomics or epidemiology. Get all the anger out, which is likely to really tire you, giving you a much better chance of finally falling asleep.

Get up when you can't sleep. If you are tossing and turning and can't get to sleep after about ten or fifteen minutes, get out of bed and go into the guest room and toss and turn on the bed there. If you don't have a guest room, go next door, briefly apologizing to your neighbors about waking them at 1 a.m. and ask if they have a guest room.

And finally, use your bed only for sleep and sex. Ideally, not at the same time.

Napping for dummies

OKAY, ALTHOUGH NAPS CAN INTERFERE WITH SLEEP AND we strongly advise against them, you're probably going to want to take them anyway, because naps feel really good. In fact, studies from the National Siesta Study have shown that 82 percent of Nobel Prize winners have taken naps. Without naps, most of us would probably just mindlessly be killing time before it's time to go to sleep.

If you're definitely going to nap—and you probably are—here's how to do it better.

Before the nap

When should you choose to take a nap? The obvious answer is "when you're tired." The obvious comeback question to the obvious answer is "when are you *not* tired?" So, then, think back to that day in February 1973, the glorious last time you slept past 7:15 in the morning.

When is the best time for napping? Some people like a morning nap, others prefer early afternoon, and there are a few people who go for one right before dinner. During dinner also can work, particularly if you want to avoid any dining table discussion of the benefits of flossing.

In fact, all these options are good, and the only way to know which is best for you is to try all of them, one after the other, on a day when you are trying to avoid cleaning out the attic or organizing your travel toothpaste collection.

Carefully choose where you are going to do your napping. You want to do it in a restful environment. You should nap, that is, in a quiet, dark place with a comfortable room temperature, and few distractions. Madison Square Garden, for example, would not be a good place even though the Knicks can easily put you to sleep. Instead, consider your kitchen pantry, unless it's full of exploding cans of expired creamed corn.

Most experts advise against napping while driving, eating, or showering. You can nap, however, while taking a bath, but be aware that if you're selling your house, your real estate agent just might pop into the bathroom with potential buyers and there goes getting the listed price.

Set an alarm before you lie down. Be sure to put it in another room so it will not disturb you.

During the nap

Do not spend your nap time thinking of what you should be doing or could be doing during your nap time. You probably wouldn't do any of it anyway and would be scrolling on Facebook instead.

Keep your nap short. If it's longer than six hours, you will be forced to rename it sleep and then where will you be?

Experts say to aim for twenty to thirty minutes. Most experts, of course, aren't nearly as tired as you are.

But you also don't want to make your nap too short. The ideal length of a nap depends, obviously, on the person, so find a person who will allow you to nap for as long as you want.

After the nap

You may feel a little groggy following a short daytime nap. That's normal. Wake yourself up with a cold shower or a hot cross bun. Do not operate complicated machinery—like the toilet—until you have cleared your head and been able to answer the Final Jeopardy question. Make sure it's in the form of a question.

If it isn't, that means you're still too groggy and probably need another nap.

Building a Better Diet

Food for thought

If we want to lengthen our lifespan, seem more youthful and help ward off the downsides of aging, such as getting older, it's not enough just to exercise more and sleep better. As we age, we also have to watch more carefully what we eat and drink. That means, in addition to much else, no more breakfasts full of Doritos, cheap beer, and other essential nutrients.

When we were younger, we could eat whatever we wanted even if all we wanted was Good 'n' Plenty. Our bodies were young and resilient enough that they could withstand an overabundance of Nestle's Crunch.

We didn't know, or care, if a certain food would help boost our immune system and another could give us scurvy. We weren't aware that apple cider vinegar is a natural laxative and that seeds and whole grains provide the necessary amount of manganese since we couldn't identify manganese in a lineup. And who wanted to eat seeds when you could get a Good Humor Creamsicle?

But as we age, our metabolism slows and is required by law to stay in the right lane. Similarly, our bodies have become less effective at absorbing important nutrients because they have forgotten if they left the nutrients in the pantry or brought them upstairs so they could chew on them while watching TV in the den.

So, we have come to the realization that eating healthy and maintaining a well-balanced diet can help us stay energized and lower the risk of developing chronic health conditions, such as heart disease, diabetes, and the relentless urge to nag our adult children. Additionally, it keeps our weight at a good level and keeps our minds sharp as a tack, unless we're asked to name the movie we saw last night.

And to eat healthy, as we are told again and again, we should consume foods rich in fiber, vitamins, minerals, and other nutrients, even if they taste like bubble wrap. We should not eat foods high in processed sugars, saturated fats and salt, no matter how much we've been dreaming of Double Stuf Oreos.

But this is not as simple as it seems. Like much else in our lives, eating has gotten complicated and has become a marathon of data overload. Before putting anything in our mouths, we are inundated with information from labels, blogs, books, YouTube videos, cable infomercials, Facebook ads, and Gwyneth Paltrow, which means we now have a lot more confusing data that we can easily misunderstand.

And thus, questions remain, like what is too much sodium

and not enough vitamin D? Does this food have gluten, and does that food have palm oil? What is gluten anyway, and who invented it eighteen years ago? Are we ingesting too much saturated fat or taking in enough Omega-3s? Why aren't there any Omega-2s? Is our calcium intake up to snuff? If not, should we consider taking snuff supplements?

Sure, one glass of red wine a day is good for you, according to some studies, but two glasses—according to other studies—maybe not so good. Or maybe it's three glasses, but not right before bedtime? Are we talking here about those really big glasses from the back of the cupboard or those fragile dinky little ones we got for a wedding present years ago and have never used? Plus, if red wine is good, is white wine bad? And how about rosé—whose side is it on?

We wonder: Will this food help our gout or worsen our goiter? Are we getting just the right amount of iron or too much riboflavin? How much magnesium does our Hershey's almond nut bar provide, and what percentage of our daily need for magnesium does it have, even if we don't know for sure if magnesium is good or bad?

Are carrots really "vitamins for the brain" and even though it may help fight cancer, why is broccoli generally tasteless unless you dunk it in sriracha sauce? And does anyone really know what beta carotene is?

It's questions like these, according to a new study in the *Annals of Intestinal Reflux*, why most Americans, particularly older ones, have given up eating food completely in favor of watching food on *The Great British Bake Off*.

The nutrition condition

WELL, YES, WE SHOULD EAT MORE OF THIS AND LESS OF that. Or maybe it's eat more of that and less of this. Whatever.

The thing is, as noted, dietary advice can be confusing. Fortunately, I can clarify and offer some general nutritional guidelines concerning common food and drink categories so you will be able to navigate dangerous times like lunch:

Wine. One glass of red wine a day is, in fact, good for you, except when you drink it for breakfast with your pancakes. Two glasses of wine, not so good. Three glasses of wine, you're not really going to care one way or the other and will definitely not be able to enunciate "this vintage prevents myocardial infarction." It's important, then, to make sure that your one glass is a really big one. Consider using a pitcher.

Of course, all this advice applies only to red wine. As for white wine, studies suggest that you can add red dye No. 34 to it to make it look like red wine if you don't mind increasing your usual daily intake of carcinogenic chemicals. (You may have to cut down on the house brand boxes of mac 'n glow-in-the-dark cheese.)

Salt. We need salt to balance our electrolytes, or else they would lose their balance and could trip and fall while walking down the stairs. Salt also helps our bodies maintain the right amount of fluid. Too much salt, however, can raise your blood pressure, endangering your heart and damaging your kidneys, neither of which has gotten good reviews on Trip Advisor.

For decades, health experts have been debating whether we should cut back on our daily salt intake. Recently, though, the Foundation for Alimentary Troubles (FART) found that the right amount of salt could either be good or bad for your health or perhaps somewhere in between. Or as they finally determined, in a meta-analysis of other analyses, who really knows?

To make sure then that you are ingesting exactly the right amount, always carry a salt shaker around with you in your pocket, preferably right-side up. And never refer to salt as sodium chloride because that's showing off and nobody likes a showoff.

Sugar. It's important to distinguish between sugars. Natural sugars are found in lots of different foods, although, unfortunately, pistachio mocha ice cream is not one of them. Their job is to keep things sweet and supply glucose to the brain and provide energy to cells around the body, even when the body would prefer napping or watching golf on TV, which is pretty much the same thing. These natural sugars are also digested more slowly, thus making you feel full for longer and, in theory, preventing you from gorging on pistachio mocha ice cream.

On the other hand, unnatural sugar, or what is called refined sugar, has been processed so often that it looks like beef jerky without the beef. Excessive consumption of refined sugar has been associated with poorer memory and something else that I can't recall. Too much refined sugar can mean empty calories (equivalent to 1.4 Euros) and can increase your risk of obesity, diabetes, and heart disease.

Then again, it might not, particularly if you are already obese and have diabetes and heart disease. It does, however, make pistachio mocha ice cream taste awfully good, so it's absolutely your call.

Fiber. Fiber can help lower cholesterol, improve heart health, and keep us regular, although it does tend to stick in your teeth. That is particularly important as our metabolism changes and we lose most of our teeth.

Fiber acts like a scrub brush for your colon, which is far superior to having to swallow a vacuum cleaner and getting it all the way down there, even if you're using one of those little hand-held ones. Fiber can be found in whole grains and legumes (from the Greek *Leguminosae*, or, in English, cardboard). Legumes include black beans, soybeans, pinto beans, kidney beans, lima beans, and other members of the bean family, even cousins, but not by marriage.

Chocolate. Depends on whom you ask. Cardiologists say that eating one Hershey's almond nut bar a day will help prevent heart disease, mainly because it has flavanols and antioxidants (although Hershey's has chosen, for reasons that are unclear, not to have named the bar Hershey's Flavanol Antioxidant Bar). Dermatologists say it will give you zits.

If you need to get a third opinion, you can always get one at Ben and Jerry's.

What you should eat

MANY OF THE DIETARY ESSENTIALS WE SHOULD BE consuming are found in what we now call superfoods. We have given them this name because Doritos was already taken. These foods are not just good for you, they also make you feel vastly superior to all those bozos at the state fair chowing down on french-fried beef jerky chips.

These superfoods, which contain no chemicals but lots of organic, minimally processed air, all have been around for a long time, but nobody paid much attention to them because they didn't go well with barbecue sauce. Then research showed they can help fight disease, extend our lifespans, and scare the daylights out of those of us already concerned about our prostates and worried about our creaky knees.

Even if they taste like talcum powder, these are the foods we boomers *should* be eating to help us live longer and still be around when Jeff Bezos buys Germany.

Apples. Full of soluble fiber, apples help reduce cholesterol. That's the bad cholesterol, obviously. Well, probably. Or maybe they increase the good cholesterol, which is either HDL, LDL, or NHL. Or it's possible they make the bad cholesterol into the good cholesterol by some alchemic process similar to how eating a chocolate chip cookie makes you forget how you promised to start dieting. Eat at least an apple a day. You know why.

Asparagus. This is a vegetable high in lycopene, which, in a double-blind study increased carotenoid levels significantly in healthy subjects who consumed shots of unadulterated lycopene on the rocks for twenty-six days in a row. Increased carotenoid levels may better protect the spleen and pancreas, whatever they are, as long as you are willing to waste twenty-six days of your life drinking unadulterated lycopene. Asparagus can be eaten grilled, steamed, sautéed, or put into your food processor and made into a juice that you will never drink because it's, you know, green.

Blueberries. Rich in antioxidants, blueberries can improve your immune system by staining it blue and thus camouflaging it from the other flesh-colored internal systems. Blueberries also boast flavonoids, which, in addition to preventing inflammation, are particularly attractive because they sound like something that might actually have flavor and so you are more likely to eat them with your Count Chocula morning cereal.

Bran. Bran is that chewy thing that has been removed from the hard outer shell of a whole grain cereal, leaving only the endosperm, which if taken to excess may leave you infertile.

Also a small village in eastern Romania, bran is full of zinc, selenium, and folate, which underpaid eastern Romanian peasants have tirelessly mined in the selenium mines for generations. Also found in heavy metals, these minerals will keep your metabolism under control but could cause problems at an airport security checkpoint. Eating a lot of bran will make you appreciate asparagus juice.

Broccoli. Broccoli is high in vitamins such as A, C, B9, B52, and C3PO. That means your eyes, red blood cells, bones, and tissues all benefit from this vegetable, but you're the one who has to taste it. Broccoli can be served either raw or cooked, though research has proven that it will still remain broccoli.

Chocolate. The antioxidants in dark chocolate have been shown to lower blood pressure, reduce the risk of clotting, and increase blood circulation to the heart, thus lowering the risks of stroke, coronary heart disease, and death from heart disease. Most important, it works a lot better in a Snickers bar than broccoli does.

Butternut squash. This is a vegetable that is brimming with potassium, which we need to keep our potassium levels at a brimming level. According to studies from the squash institute, if you eat one butternut squash a day for the next six and a half years, you're going to be really tired of butternut squash.

Fava beans. Low in fat, low in sodium, and low in flavor, these beans have plenty of manganese and iron, which is what probably makes them taste so awful. Their inability to be easily digested will help keep your weight down. The good news about fava beans? They're not as tasteless as lima beans.

Garbanzos. Bursting with protein, copper, and zinc, garbanzos—also known as chick peas after they were placed in a legume protection program—are extremely versatile and can ruin a salad or a stew.

Mangoes. Just a cup of mangoes supplies more than 10 percent of a day's requirement of vitamin A and around two-thirds of a day's requirement of vitamin C. Researchers are still trying to determine why it just skipped over vitamin B for apparently no reason.

Nuts. A dense source of nutrients, nuts promote brain and heart health as long as you remember to take the shells off before swallowing. Nuts provide important minerals like vitamin E, calcium and selenium, unless they never get into your digestive system because they are stuck in your teeth.

And of course, it's important to remember to always eat and drink all these superfoods in moderation, except, obviously, for fava beans, where one is more than enough.

Weight, weight, don't tell me

During the recent period of prolonged isolation and abundant Cheetos, have you been gaining weight, despite focusing on eating superfoods? Have you noticed your pants getting tighter?

This may be happening because we still are trying to wear the bell-bottoms we wore to that 1975 Barry Manilow concert. But it's probably equally likely we've gained some weight because of an aging metabolism.

Metabolism is the sum of the chemical reactions in the body's cells that changes food into energy, Metabolism slows as we get older so sometimes it can barely get out the door in time for a 2 p.m. urologist appointment. We could speed up our metabolism by using higher octane, but who wants to get to a urologist's office too early?

Then there's the problem of calories. According to numbers from the U.S. Department of Numbers, on an average day the average person should take in an average of 2,000 calories. But that doesn't include the senior discount!

Without the discount, boomers can gain lots of weight, which can lead to increased risk of heart disease and the inability to fit through a revolving door. Plus, it may mean you have to get rid of those bell bottoms, or at least wear them upside down.

So, if you've taken in too many calories and want to lose a few pounds, there's always the option of taking in fewer calories. Of course, that may be too complicated a solution for many of us who want to lose eight pounds this afternoon before going out for dinner tonight with friends we haven't seen since high school.

Instead, you could always follow one of these popular dieting plans:

The Mediterranean Diet. This is a way of eating based on the traditional cuisine of countries bordering the Mediterranean Sea. These include Italy, Greece, and Spain, but not New Jersey. The diet typically consists of the region's fruits, vegetables, and seafood, doused in so much olive oil you can't distinguish among them. The premium version of the diet includes an all-expense-paid trip to a Greek island and a stay at an Airbnb where the hosts are extra virgins.

The Paleo Diet. This is a plan based on foods similar to what might have been eaten during the Paleolithic era, which dates from approximately 2.5 million to 10,000 years ago, so check the "best by" dates closely.

The idea behind the diet is that if you could hunt and gather it, you can eat it. That means yes to meats, fruits, and veggies, but no to Devil Dogs, caramel popcorn, and Good 'n' Plenty, unless you have a license to hunt Good 'n' Plenty during its fall breeding season.

Although research isn't conclusive, one small study has found that after three weeks on this diet subjects had dropped an average of five pounds, mainly by tearing their hair out.

The South Beach Diet. Named after a glamorous area of Miami, which will be fully under water by the time you are done with this diet, this is sometimes called a modified low-carbohydrate plan. It is lower in carbs and higher in sand than other, more inland diets.

On this fiber-rich diet, you can eat all the complex carbs you want, including fruit, vegetables, whole grains, beans, and legumes. Unfortunately, you may still be very hungry and dying for a Baby Ruth.

The Low-Fat, High-Carb Diet. When you sit down at the table, divide your food into those with a minimal amount of fat, like celery stalks and facial tissues, which you put on the left. High-carb foods, like white bread, pasta, and toothpaste, you put on the right. Stare at both piles, then pull up pictures of Twinkies on your smartphone and begin to salivate, thus losing any water-weight gain.

The High-Fat, Low-Carb Diet. This is exactly like what the Low-Fat, High-Carb Diet looks like when it is staring at a mirror. Sometimes known as the Keto diet, this eating plan relies on using up ketone bodies, the fuel your liver produces from the fat it has been storing pointlessly for years. After a few days on this diet, your body will reach the state of ketosis, unless you have made a wrong turn and ended up in Kentucky. Next time, use the GPS!

The Good 'n' Plenty Diet. For breakfast, eat the white ones first, then the pink ones. For lunch, work in the opposite direction, balancing your intake. For dinner, gobble them both up at the same time. You may not lose weight, but you'll make your dentist happy.

⇒ *Update Alert* ⇐

As we head into the remainder of this book, we need to install a new operating system for the complicated, highly technical tech section. Please do not close the book during the process.

Yes, we know this is not fair to us boomers who grew up thinking the IBM Selectric was the ultimate in technological innovation. Yes, we do understand that some in our age cohort have only just learned how to change a voicemail greeting without deleting all previous voice mails. And yes, we get how many of us feel about complex new technology allegedly designed to make our lives simpler while, actually, making us feel dumber than an analog.

But becoming a better boomer means making adjustments, even if we have to call the kids again and ask them to explain to us one more time how all this works, including what's the real purpose of the F8 key on the laptop, whether you can use airplane mode if you're stuck in basic economy, and is encryption as creepy as we think it is?

And please understand, this is our first new operating system in several chapters and we felt it was needed even though the old operating system worked perfectly well and at least some of us had really mastered it.

Although the new operating system has been designed to eliminate all previous glitches, such as paper cuts while turning pages, particularly on your Kindle, there are sure to be some new glitches. (In fact, GLITCH is now the name of our new holding company [NYSE: GLTH], which, after our IPO, is already valued at $74 billion.) Consequently, we suggest you back up any files that come anywhere near this book. This includes irreplaceable items you have held on to like last month's grocery receipts or your handwritten to-do list from December 2012.

The new operating system we will be using, update 8.02.4/6, designed to replace update 8.02.4/5, which replaced 8.02.4/4, offers an all-new design and all-new features, none of which you will be able to easily understand or operate. Which is, after all, the whole point of a new operating system, isn't it?

The new system will enable improvements in usability and security and will sync with all your old Beatles records. All functionalities will be simplified, but nevertheless may still be called functionalities.

Thanks to new facial recognition software, this new operating system will allow you to be able to laugh occasionally without even having to read any words—just stare at the pages and guffaws will come pouring out. (As a bonus, the facial recognition software does not recognize receding hairlines or deeply embedded wrinkles.) Just a passing glance at the cover will provide a few chuckles. A momentary glimpse will get you a couple of snickers. By pressing control-alt-~ or delete-shift-&, you will be able to immediately control yourself when you start to laugh so loudly you are disturbing the neighbors.

With the new operating system, if you need to find a particularly clever play on words, just quickly access our new word playlist and find puns, jests, quips, witticisms, gags, wisecracks, and, if you have unlimited data, maybe even some jokes. (Some of the jokes may be available offline, but only if you have memorized certain sections.)

The new operating system comes with built-in nouns, some verbs, and occasional prepositions, plus completely free access to the adverb store if you need it. You will probably need it.

Before you install the system, make sure you have backed up all your essential personal data because it's likely all of it will disappear into thin air during the process and wind up on some hacker's screen in Tajikistan.

When you are ready to load the system, click on "download" or "update now" or "over here, dummy." It's the big blue button in the center. However, it's also possible it might be the green button near the bottom.

Good. There are now 81 more updates to be installed to get to the full new operating system. While they happen, watch a ballgame or complain about Update No. 16.

Finally, before the new operating system is fully installed, remember to attest that you are not a robot. If you are in fact a robot, good for you. That means you may be able to understand all of this and also not have to worry about fallen arches or high cholesterol levels.

After you have completed the installation, take a nap because you will be exhausted. When you awake, we hope you will appreciate all our hard work and are willing to give us at least four stars on Yelp.

Building a Better Techie

Digital overload

We grew up in an age of transistor radios. It was a time of limited technological choice—the transistor radios could get only three AM stations and two of them were playing Ferrante and Teicher's theme from *Exodus*.

If we wanted to look something up, we went to the *Encyclopedia Britannica*, which our parents had bought on the installment plan (a kind of early Venmo), and was sort of like Wikipedia but weighed more, and volume Tar-Vew didn't have a hyperlink to volume Mou-Nyo.

Our information screens were limited to three television channels, all of which seemed to be showing *Bonanza* when they weren't showing *Have Gun—Will Travel*. Alexa was not yet a virtual assistant nor the name of the girl sitting behind us in third grade. That was Carol or Marion or Joan (Sidney was still a boy's name). We also had landlines, although they weren't yet called landlines because they didn't need a first name since they were the only lines we had.

New technology was mom's recently purchased toaster, the one with four (!) different settings, including burnt.

Today our low-technology generation is awash in high-tech and we are struggling to stay afloat, not to mention connected. Inundated by a plethora of gadgets and gizmos, we are overwhelmed with remote-controlled contraptions and multitasking thingamajigs, which, of course, can only be connected wirelessly, assuming you have the right doohickey.

We have surrounded ourselves with a whole new cohort of assistants, who do things we hadn't known needed doing. Alongside Alexa, there's Siri and Cortana, Nest and Echo, the Vitamix and the Spiralizer, Bluetooth and Blu-ray, Fitbits and Kindles, Glipsies and Shmaltzers. (I may have made those last two up, although I'm not quite sure.)

Now, in addition, we have the growth of AI, artificial intelligence, with bots like ChatGPT, which can do almost everything a human brain can do except explain artificial intelligence so some of us can understand it.

All this technology has insinuated itself into our daily lives, supposedly simplifying everything we do. But, c'mon. In reality, of course, it complicates everything.

We now have to program, or try to program, the electric tea kettle. We must fiddle with adjusting the sleep number of our bed even when napping on the couch. We try to access the house thermostat through our phone when we are thousands of miles away from home and can't look out the window to see if it is raining there. When we return home, we find we've set the temperature to 91 degrees in the living room and it is snowing in the kitchen.

Trying to buy a new car, we are intimidated by the dashboard technology display, which looks like CNBC updates on how the Dow Jones Industrials are faring. How can you concentrate on driving and cutting off the guy in the next lane when you are also carefully watching the digital read-out of your GPS directions, tire pressure, air-fuel ratio, battery strength, rear-end camera view, side camera view, and of course the satellite radio receiver playing classic soft rock and scrolling Simon and Garfunkel lyrics?

Even purchasing a new pair of sneakers, you need to get your foot digitally scanned, the data from the scan is fed into an algorithm, then it's graphed onto a database, and then you are quickly told you owe $149.95 *for a pair of sneakers*.

We feel overloaded with digital data, pinged to exasperation. Our watches now don't just tell us the time, they tell us our heart rate, how many miles we've run, how many steps we've taken, how many calories expended, how many hours we've slept—or, more accurately, not slept—and then (this is true) my watch has the nerve to tell me I'm too stressed and should take a few deep breaths to calm myself. Of course, I'm too stressed—I'm way behind on my step count.

We all have been conditioned through these new technological innovations to expect immediate results, instant communication, abundant choices, gratification without delay.

The problem is, our generation had grown used to delayed gratification. We had waited, after all, nine years for the Vietnam War to finally stop. We had waited for the Captain and Tennille to end. For tofu and Richard Simmons and disco to go away. We have waited for our kids to finally give us grandchildren, for joy without responsibility.

Newer generations expect to microwave dinner in a few minutes, find the name of the best Asian fusion restaurant in downtown Indianapolis in a few seconds, receive a response to an urgent text right now, and be able to check their Insta this instant. We, on the other hand, had always sent birthday cards that might arrive next week, only three days after the birthday (but only if we had remembered to actually lick the stamp). We had waited for the morning newspaper, when there was a morning paper, which was made of actual paper, to tell us what had happened yesterday. And if that wasn't current enough, we waited for the evening news, which would be on in just another seven hours or so, when Walter Cronkite could tell us what had happened earlier today.

We could wait to call a friend back because we didn't know the friend had called us since there was no voice mail on which to leave a message. We could wait for the pot to boil and not get exasperated that it wasn't an Instant Pot or when the microwave took twenty seconds, not fifteen.

We were so used to waiting we actually had come to embrace the idea of cliffhangers and were reasonably OK with not immediately knowing who shot JR. We could wait until next season to find out it was all a dream and that it wasn't either the Captain or Tennille who had shot him.

Now, when we're trying to think, for instance, of the capital of Montana—although I'm not sure why we would ever want to know the capital of Montana—we Google and immediately (0.66 seconds, 3,040,000 results) find out, yes, it's still Helena. We have lost the ultimate boomer thrill of saying, "Oh, I'm not going to be able to sleep tonight unless I can think of what that is." (Of course, that generally was easy to say, since most of us don't sleep very well.)

Getting the answer so quickly keeps us from the reassuring sense that it's right there, on the tip of our tongues, and if we just had a little more time or could concentrate a little more effectively or perhaps if we had a shorter tongue, we could definitely get it.

Trying to come up with the answer, by ourselves, has been a kind of boomer intellectual calisthenic that was definitely going to make our brains work harder. Searching for the name, we'd be stimulating new connections between nerve cells and helping develop more neurological plasticity and building up a functional reserve that would provide a hedge against future cell loss as we age. Right?

On the other hand, 0.66 seconds does seem awfully attractive even if we first have to look at the sponsored list of the top ten Asian fusion restaurants in downtown Helena.

Between two worlds

So, YES, MOST OF THE TIME, WE DO GOOGLE THE ANSWER. We do scan our timeline. Of course, we GPS the trip and check our texts and post our pix. We prefer to nuke rather than cook. We FaceTime rather than drop over. We open the weather app rather than look out the window.

Yet many of us still own a VCR and a number of audio cassettes, maybe a subscription to a print newspaper, or have a car that you actually unlock with an actual key. And occasionally we may even listen to ballgames on AM radio because we still have an AM radio.

We are a generation, that is, caught between two worlds, stuck between ChatGPT and Betamax VHS. And such a fondness for the past, in the midst of the digital present, can be problematic. It is, after all, hard to send emails from our Underwood manual typewriter or insert carbon paper into our computer printer. Not to mention the difficulties of running with a Walkman.

With one foot firmly planted in earlier decades, many of us have difficulty planting the other foot into the present. It's why we want to have the new whatchamacallit but struggle with how it works and whether it is different from the last whatchamacallit. It's why many of us are still unable to tell the difference between a doohickey and a dongle.

By the way, if you're interested: A doohickey is a term used in a vague way to refer to something whose name one cannot recall, like that . . . thing. However, a dongle is a small piece of computer hardware that connects to a port on another device to provide it with additional functionality, or enable a pass-through to such a device that adds functionality. Yeah, that doesn't make any sense.

As an example, I recently bought a new washing machine. Like smartphones, fitness watches, personal voice assistants, wifi extenders, and digital meat thermometers, it had a number of unfathomable doohickeys and a bunch of complicated whatchamacallits. Unfortunately, what it didn't have, like most new technology, was clear, intelligible directions for those of us from the transistor radio generation on how to install it and operate it.

But I did learn a few things all of us need to know about new technology.

Don't waste time searching for the manual. There is never a physical manual in the box accompanying your machine or device, so this is time that could be better spent complaining about how difficult it is to open the box.

When you finally do get the box opened, inside you may find a number of Apple decals, advertisements for high-tech laundry detergent (but not if you've bought a new phone), several small desiccant packs, and lots of bubble wrap. But there's no manual because you are supposed to go online to check out the manual.

This, of course, assumes you can view the 82-page "Easy Start-up" online manual, if you have already set up an online account, created a user name and password, and agreed to receive three online newsletters and advertisements per day.

Check the language of the instruction manual. When you finally do get to the instruction manual, do not follow the Mandarin-language directions unless you are Mandarin.

Don't waste time calling the customer help line. Even though you are well aware that your call is important to them, it's always good to remember that it's not nearly as important to them as it is to you because, frankly, they're a robot voice created by artificial intelligence and they have all the time in the world and never have to go to the bathroom or search for a Nutty Buddy Bar.

Don't be fooled by instructional illustrations. These are not necessarily obscene, but then again, who really knows? These are usually very ambiguous tiny line drawings obviously drawn by someone's particularly precocious grandchild. They are so small and unclear you may think they are telling you to plug Cable C into the USB port when they are really telling you to put on tactical hazard gear.

Beware live chats. You may be encouraged to do a live

chat if you cannot figure out where the USB port is, where to put the dongle, or if you're still having difficulty opening the box. It's important here to note that the person with whom you may be doing a live chat is not, in fact, a person. Nor live.

It is a robot programmed to keep you from calling *Consumer Reports* and giving your new device only a 2.5-star review.

Know the limits of your tech skills. Installing, for instance, a new Dual Band Gigabit ADSL+ 2.4 and 5 Ghz wireless modem/router (and I only wish I was making up that name) by yourself is probably beyond your capability. (Deciding what the differences were among "cool," "cold" and "tap cold" on my new Zeph-200-G stainless steel washing machine was easily beyond my capability).

Never forget there are alternatives. For instance, you could completely give up all the tech, live off the land, and become an off-the-grid hermit in a Wyoming cave, but only if you have an extremely unlimited data plan.

And, fortunately, if all else fails, you can always play with the bubble wrap.

What's the word?

THE MOST DIFFICULT PART OF ADAPTING TO THE NEW high-tech world if you're at least partly an old-tech person? Or if you're just old?

The answer, obviously, must be at least eight characters long, include a capital and a lower-case letter, a number, a symbol, maybe even a cheese Danish, and make no sense at all. In other words, a password.

We now need them for pretty much everything we do, every connection we try to make. They are the indispensable signature of the high-tech age, required for ordering from Amazon, checking our bank balance, communicating with friends, or posting snide comments about friends on multiple platforms. They are obligatory for accessing our credit card accounts, signing into our tax preparer's ultra-secret portal, and ignoring emails from estranged relatives. They are our connection to the news, to shopping, and to our private notes on our personal blood pressure readings.

Passwords, we are relentlessly assured, are designed to protect us. And we need that protection because as boomers, supposedly not as familiar with high-tech gadgetry and the online world, we are considered to be at particular risk for fraud and identity theft. We are more susceptible to scams and criminality, in case anyone wants to illicitly use the fact we've bought argyle compression socks on Amazon or wants our personal blood pressure readings.

Online security is important because we live in a time when identity theft has continued to grow. In fact, according to the most recent estimate, someone's identity is stolen every three minutes, but because of our new privacy regulations we are not permitted to identify that someone. It's possible it may be your Pilates instructor, but we can't be sure.

So, we need passwords. But remembering all those passwords is difficult. Unlike younger people, our heads are already filled with detritus like the starting lineup for the 1955 Brooklyn Dodgers and the name of the group that sang "Leader of the Pack." Despite trying to shove them out of the way, we have never forgotten the entire Castro Convertible TV commercial jingle and the last line of dialogue from the movie (not the remake!) *Invasion of the Body Snatchers.*

[The answers in order: Junior Gilliam, Pee Wee Reese, Duke Snider, Gil Hodges, Sandy Amoros, Jackie Robinson, Carl Furillo, Roy Campanella; The Shangri-Las; "Who conquered space with fine design? Who saves you money all the time? Who's tops in the convertible line? Castro

Convertible!"; and "Operator, get me the Federal Bureau of Investigation. Yes, it's an emergency."]

Yet we have difficulty remembering which is the bank password and which is the one for the health portal at the urologist's office. We can't keep track of what to use for Netflix, and what's the one for our health insurance account? Does the password for our Delta Airlines frequent flyer account have a space between the street address number we used and the street? Is the credit card password the one that ends with the $% or is that the utility company?

Yes, we could use something called a password manager, which would keep track of all our passwords, but then we'd have to figure out how to use something called a password manager.

Like many boomers forced to deal with overtaxed memory capacity, at first I tried to keep the passwords as simple as possible, so I'd at least have a chance at recalling them. That is, I started out using the same password for all my accounts. It was a password I knew well and was unlikely to forget. It was my first name.

I thought it was perfect—a heady mixture of vowels and consonants. It used *both* a capital letter and a few lowercase ones. Most important, I was usually able to remember it. But then everyone—what I mean by that is my wife—kept telling me my password concept was too simple and not safe. It didn't have at least eight characters. And it didn't have any symbols or numbers or Romanian acronyms.

Passwords shouldn't be something any hacker could easily figure out. Let's make them earn their hack!

Here, then, are some recommendations I've learned on how to create—and how to remember!—the perfect password, which, by the way, you will need to continue reading the remainder of this book. Without a password, you will be blocked by the firewall, which we have installed between pages 134 and 136 and can be removed only by certified Geek Squad technicians.

Do not use the same password for multiple accounts. You don't want to make an appointment at your urologist's office by mistake and find out you have a high prostate number when you had planned to get a reservation for two, on the patio, at that nice new Italian seafood place. Once hackers can determine your urologist password, they may get unnecessarily concerned about their own endocrine levels.

Take a sentence and turn it into a password. Select a phrase or a song lyric or a book title that's particularly memorable to you, such as Now Is The Time for All Good Men to Come to the Aid of Their Country or That's Why I Fell for the Leader of the Pack. Take the first letter of each word in the sentence (for instance, TWIFftLotP) and create your password.

Then always include a Cyrillic number, such as **✗aѰs.** Be sure not to confuse that with **✗зр̄йi**.

Make sure your password includes an umlaut. If you do not know what an umlaut is, or the umlaut store is simply out of them, they can be replaced temporarily with a **~**.

Choose a series of unrelated common words. This could be something like *cloud tomato, acrylic Beyonce,* or *political integrity.*

Use a series of numbers in your password. These should be random numbers. It's really best if they aren't 1234567890. Trust me.

Your password cannot be the same as your user name. Unless, of course, your user name is 1234567890.

And finally, and this may go without saying—but, you know—never use the word *password* as your password. Not even p@ssword, unless you add an umlaut.

Call for security

Unfortunately, it's not always enough just to have a complex, inscrutable password when you want to check your email or access your bank account or buy a bottle of anti-aging repairing eye stick from an online retailer. Just to be extra sure you are who you say you are and not a hacker from Moldova—unless you are, in fact, a hacker from Moldova—you also may have to answer a few security questions.

This is because passwords, even inscrutable ones, are sometimes not sufficient to safeguard your accounts and protect your identity from being stolen and maybe observed out on the street embarrassingly wearing brown shoes with white socks. Just recently, in fact, a prominent password manager app was itself hacked, exposing thousands of passwords who had been minding their own business and telling each other jokes with punchlines ending in #$%J3! Frankly, I didn't get the joke, but that may just be me.

So, in addition to passwords, we have security questions. Of course, we set up those security questions years ago, never realizing we might have to answer them years later, after our brains had been stuffed with so much extraneous detail, like the results of 1984 preseason NFL games and recipes for Swedish meatballs. The answers, which seemed obvious at the time, may not come as easily now, particularly to those of us who have difficulty recalling what we ate for dinner last night or where we live.

Remember, then, if you're setting up security questions and answers today, don't depend on unverifiable, misty recollections. When my wife was asked recently, after inputting her password, *who was your childhood best friend?* her immediate response was Caroline, because that's the only old friend with whom she's still in touch. But the answer turned out to be Valerie, because Valerie's mother was the one who had given her mother the recipe for Swedish meatballs.

There are ways to avoid these problems. If you're setting up security questions and answers today, remember this:

Don't depend on unverifiable and thus potentially variable responses. You may have once put down your dream vacation destination as Paris, but what if the Parisians really piss you off now with their snooty ways and the price of baguettes has hit the roof? Today you might answer Florida, which is always a mistake.

Never use searchable real answers to the security questions. Hackers who have done their homework can easily know what city you were born in and your mother's maiden name. Instead of the real answers, create ones that only have meaning to you. As an example, if you are asked your mother's maiden name, respond Baguette.

If you insist on using your mother's real maiden name, tattoo it on your arm. Put a tattoo on your hand so you'll remember which arm.

And obviously never admit that your first car was a Ford Pinto.

Don't try to show off. When the security question is *What is your favorite book?*, don't try to snow them by responding *War and Peace*, which, you know, you never actually finished, when the real answer is the most recent schlock by Danielle Steel or the sequel to the sequel of 50 *Shades of Grey*.

Make it memorable. The answer to the question should immediately pop into your head, even if you're logging in years after you first created the account. For instance, you could use the name of your first pet unless you never had a first pet because of all those allergies, or at least that's what your parents told you because they didn't want to be bothered.

And most important, remember that *you* will get only a couple of chances to answer the security questions correctly before you are shut out from the account and have to go to Moldova and search for it there.

Terms of endearment

Do you ever get the feeling that everybody—particularly those who are digital natives or just, say, younger than our socks—is speaking a different language than we boomers? I suppose it could be French or Spanish. But it's probably emoji.

In fact, they are tech talking, using words, phrases, acronyms, and secret signals that show off how utterly up-to-date and hip they are and how utterly un-up-to-date and un-hip the rest of us are.

Yes, we sometimes do need a glossary to figure out exactly what they are talking about. Luckily, here's one.

AI. These initials stand for artificial intelligence, which is the ability of a computer to do tasks that are usually done by humans. Unfortunately, these tasks never include flossing.

Algorithm. Al got rhythm, Al got music, Al got my gal, who could ask for anything more?

Bandwidth. When your adult children say they are too busy with their PTA meetings, book clubs, garage bands, or something on Netflix, they will explain the reason they didn't call and wish Aunt Mildred happy birthday on Sunday was because they were exhausted and "didn't have enough bandwidth."

Bluetooth. Probably not a sign of bad dental hygiene, or lack of flossing, but, instead, a wireless communications technology intended to replace a cable. And who doesn't want to replace Spectrum or Comcast?

Browser. Just looking.

The cloud. A mysterious place way high above that somehow keeps track of all your data and the pictures you took on that trip to Paris. Could be cirrus, but most likely cumulus.

Cookie. A piece of code or data created and left on a user's computer unless it is homemade chocolate chip, which is never left anywhere.

CPU. How you help toilet train your young grandchild.

Driver. Could be Adam, for all we know.

Encryption. To protect our communications from prying eyes, they are put into snug crypts, used for burials, which are then placed underground and gloomily reappear only during Mark Zuckerberg's scary testimony to Congress.

GIF. Technically, Graphics Interchange Format. Not so technically, GIFs are little video snippets that are generally used to make fun of boomers online by younger generations who have no idea what carbon paper is.

Hard drive. Washington to New York. Jersey Turnpike.

Influencer. Someone who has the power to affect the purchasing decisions of others because of perceived authority, knowledge, position, or relationship with his or her audience. Also, someone we've usually never heard of.

JPEG. A file format created by the Joint Photographic Experts Group, thus the name, which has become the common format used for photos displayed on the internet. It just beat out the Shared Hi-tech Item Team, fortunately.

Megabyte. Many bytes.

Megahertz. Many hertzes.

Meme. Not pronounced me-me. But you knew that, right?

RAM. Not the same as ROM.

ROM. Different from RAM.

Virtual Reality. So much better than real reality because it doesn't have pandemics, occasional lower back pain, or linoleum in the kitchen that's peeling and needs to be replaced.

WEP. I have no idea.

WPA. I have no idea.

Zip. I have zip idea.

Anti-Social

Even if we're not tech savvy, social media nevertheless has become a big part of our boomer lives, the most essential tech component, particularly during the COVID pandemic. In a time of dislocation and isolation, social media brought the world closer, as hand-in-virtual-hand we study funny cat videos together and conspire to exchange completely false information about utterly everything.

Social media is how we communicate today with our children and grandchildren, with distant colleagues and nearby neighbors. It's how we find out the latest epidemiological news and argue over the latest epidemiological news. It's a source for advice and a megaphone for opinions.

It's how we share images of our car trip to Maine that ended in Trenton, NJ, and get jealous when distant relatives are sharing images of their all-inclusive cruise to Santorini. It's how we learn of birthdays and anniversaries of those who never even registered a "like" for our birthday and anniversary post. It's how we get status updates, photos, videos, and links from people we've never met or even heard of but consider "friends." It's how we comment on subjects we know nothing about to people who know even less.

Plus, have we mentioned the funny cat videos?

For our boomer generation, social media has grown enormously because you don't need to be in the same room to actually hear what somebody is saying, even when the water is running. It gives us a chance to be friends again with people whom we knew in high school, didn't particularly care much for back then, and have avoided for the past fifty or so years. It allows us to get the word out that we've done well with today's Wordle because we're pretty sure everyone really wants to know.

Yes, admittedly, social media can be a total waste of time. Then, on the negative side, it's also addictive and destructive.

But whether we like it not, whether we understand how it works or not, it's here to stay.

As someone not on Facebook, nor Instagram, TikTok, LinkedIn, Snapchat, YouTube, Reddit or any of the others, I feel completely qualified to offer you advice on how to deal with social media and make the best of it.

Social media "friends" are not necessarily actual friends. Most likely, they would quickly report you to authorities if they believed you were cooking meth in your basement. Unless they were cooking meth in their basement.

Ignore negative posts. When someone says something nasty on social media about you or your cat, pay no attention. Of course, that kind of decent attitude will not work, and the nastiness will fester inside of you so much you will be tempted to create a false Twitter identity and profile so you can say, in response, so's your old man.

Don't worry about FOMO. FOMO is fear of missing out, a common social media malady. It's a sense that your peers are doing better than you are or have more than you do or understood what FOMO meant before you did. When we see others' pictures of spectacular vacation cruises, attendance at elegant parties, or reports about their winning the Nobel Peace Prize, naturally we may be a bit jealous. It's always important to remember then that Henry Kissinger, while he was in charge of bombing the crap out of Cambodia, won the Nobel Peace Prize.

Be careful about accepting friend requests. Don't accept any requests from people you knew many years ago in high school, particularly if you felt they may have cheated on trigonometry tests then. Those are the kind of people who could be cooking meth in their basement today.

Don't get into political arguments on social media. The reason is obvious: the people you may be arguing with will be wrong.

Find alternative activities. If you are spending too much time on social media and worry that you are becoming addicted, try replacing it with an activity that is more enjoyable for you, like screaming.

Don't succumb to pressure. There's no need to constantly update your Facebook friends or Twitter followers on interesting things you are doing if you are not doing any interesting things. Not everyone is fortunate enough to be abducted for ransom by Somali pirates.

And please, never post a cute cat video. Some of us are allergic.

Ask Mr. Techie

According to the Boomer Research and Cabana Center, 64 percent of us may still believe a tablet is something you swallow. Seventy-one percent of us still confuse a dongle with a dingle. In an increasingly digital world, it's easy to be overwhelmed by the complexities of the huge variety of devices and associated mysterious networks.

Where can you turn? Well, here.

I was born before the high-tech explosion and only recently figured out that Blu-ray was not a Darth Vader weapon. Now I'm even more confused. I am not sure if someone who uses Twitter should be considered a tweeter or a twitterer, an X-Man or a twit. Please advise.

Dear Confused:

Someone who uses the social media app known as

Twitter (or X) is someone, first of all, who in the past had to restrict his or her comments to no more than 140 characters. Now, however, thanks to improvements in biochemistry and diesel fuels, that person is now allowed to use 280 charac

---

I'm frustrated. My adult children don't answer the phone when I call them. They don't respond to emails. Now they have unfriended me on Facebook, blocked me on Instagram and don't even reply when I text them. How can you communicate with younger people today?

Dear Frustrated:

Please understand that younger people today are quite busy taking selfies (often of themselves) and creating designer pickles and craft beer made from organically sourced whey, although we don't know why. They are so caught up in today they don't want to be disturbed by yesterday's technology.

So, if it's an emergency—for instance, you really need help with figuring out whether you should use an accent mark when typing the word *anime* or you want to be sure how to pronounce GIF (hard G, soft G?)—you might try using the more millennial-oriented Snapchat or Gen Z favorite Signal to get in touch. But of course, that's only if you know which is Snapchat and which one is Signal and are certain neither is Messenger.

If nothing else works, as a last resort, you might just overnight FedEx them a sad-faced emoji. (To find the correct one, look it up at the Emojipedia. Yes, there is an Emojipedia.)

Be sure you don't send the emoji to their landline. Which, of course, they don't have.

I am concerned that I haven't backed up any of my files since 1997. I understand I could lose my documents, my contacts, my photos and my mind if something went wrong. I want to save everything to the cloud, but I don't know how to do that.

Dear Concerned:

First you have to choose your cloud. As previously noted, we recommend cumulus. Although we've seen good reviews on Yelp and Trip Advisor for cirrus.

After you make that choice, then carefully hold your laptop or mobile device (also known as your phone) above your head and up to the sky and, magically, everything gets copied to the cloud because, frankly, how else could it happen? Yes, it's a miracle.

I am worried about online security. What if someone—you know, the Russians—hacks my email accounts, discovers that I actually have responded to spam from a Nigerian prince, and steals my identity? How can I protect myself while online?

Dear Worried:

The first thing to do is change your passwords. That's always the first thing we say to do because it's so amusing to think of you trying to figure out a new password that's not a variation of an old password and then betting on whether you'll remember it.

If changing your password doesn't work, then change your user name, although you will most likely never remember which user name you should be using for which password with which site and will have to click on that little button by the sign-in box that says, "Forgot Your User Name? What an Idiot You Are."

Worst-case scenario: Your identity does get stolen and someone else, therefore, is responsible for choosing the next book for your book club, by Tuesday, or picking up the drapes at the drycleaner, or remembering to take your thyroid pill in the morning, *before* breakfast.

Not so terrible, huh?

My laptop says I should not shut it down until it finishes 143 more updates. I'm a risk-taker and want to see what could happen if I did shut it down before it is finished updating. Should I?

Dear Risk-Taker:

Although there's an undeniable thrill that comes with sticking it to the man, even if the man is really tiny and is working selflessly for digital peanuts inside your CPU, the perils of not completing your updates can be significant. You could corrupt your operating system and you could lose data and be prosecuted to the full extent of the law.

In other words, go for it. And then tell us what happened when they allow you that one phone call.

I am overwhelmed with passwords. I have too many and keep using the wrong ones. I don't even know if this is the right password that will allow me to ask you questions.

Dear Overwhelmed:

It seems your password is fine, but you have keyed in the wrong user name. Please try again.

Building a Better Retirement

Is there life after work?

EVEN WITH COVID, THE AVERAGE AMERICAN LIFESPAN is still seventy-seven years, which is an increase of almost two years from just a few decades ago and more than enough extra time to catch up on all the episodes of *The Big Bang Theory* that you might have missed when you were younger but were working a forty-hour week.

It's important to remember here that back as recently as the 1960s, when life expectancy was shorter and there was no *Big Bang Theory*, there was precious little time between when we stopped working and when we stopped living. There was also precious little to do during that time.

In those limited years available to retirees, nobody had yet invented Wordle. Plus, there was no streaming and everybody was pretty much stuck with Uncle Miltie or *The Honeymooners*.

Far worse, retirees were officially required to wear polyester leisure suits, sometimes even in the shower (they were, after all, drip-dry). You had to golf, despite not knowing a sand wedge from a sandwich. You had to interrupt your children's conversations—your children, that is, who now would be us—about the Grateful Dead by asking if their obituary had made it into the afternoon newspaper.

That was then, when there actually was an afternoon newspaper. Now, because many of us finally have gotten enough sleep and taken good care of our bodies by seeing our podiatrist regularly and drinking kombucha and increasing our dietary fiber (even though it tastes like manila folder) while sweating on the elliptical, we are far more likely to live a pretty long time without having to, you know, work. Hey, and wasn't that the original plan?

Of course, we understand not everyone can do this. Some of us boomers will continue working past a certain standard age because we have to. Some of us will continue working because we want to. And some of us will continue working because it's better than staying home, playing dominoes, acting cranky, and shouting loudly at the TV that the commercials are too loud.

But for many of us, we may finally be at the point where we don't *have* to work anymore—plus, as a bonus, we're still alive!

In other words, we can be—what's that word I'm looking for here?—retired.

In fact, according to the Leisure Suits Research Bureau, the number of retired workers receiving Social Security benefits increased from approximately 34.59 million in 2010 to

46.33 million in 2020. That accounts for, among much else, the growth of Silver Sneakers classes, erectile dysfunction drugs, and Florida.

Many new retirees had been looking forward to retirement from the moment we started working, mainly when we were stuck in traffic. This would be, we thought, the time we could do anything we wanted, if only we could figure out what we wanted.

Yet according to the National Institutes of Institutes, only 19 boomers out of the entire 46.33 million had actually planned for retirement. This happened despite all the magazine articles and TV commercials shouting at us about how to plan for retirement and the seven common mistakes to avoid in retirement planning or the five key retirement planning tips you shouldn't miss or the nine retirement blunders you shouldn't make.

The point of all this shouting was simple: retirement today doesn't just happen. If it did, you might wind up in a leisure suit in the shower. You can't just order retirement from Amazon or pick it up at the pizza place. Well, maybe you can order it from Amazon. But only if you have Prime.

Retirement planning has to start way before actual retirement. It has to be prepared for, scheduled, organized, structured, and formulated. Retirement is a lot of work, which is probably why we wait until we're not working anymore to do it.

Laying the groundwork

As you formulate your retirement plan, you need to consider some important questions first.

- Exactly when can you retire?
- When should you begin saving for retirement?
- How much money should you save?
- How much is enough, particularly if you've always been a profligate spendthrift and now have that title on your LinkedIn profile and officially embossed on your business card?
- Should you buy long-term-care insurance?
- When should you begin to think about downsizing?
- Should you retire early or wait until you can barely walk to the kitchen to get a can of seltzer?

- Do you need a retirement hobby (does snoring count?)?
- When should you take your Social Security and what about those Social Security forms—black pen or blue pen?
- Now that you have more time, do you ever intend to clean up the garage?
- Is the Required Minimum Distribution the name of a cult band that plays electronic dance music?
- Should you buy a condo in Florida? If so, which coast? Or should you just wait for more sea-level rise when there will only be one coast?
- Should you consider moving closer to the kids, even if they live in Cleveland?
- Especially if they live in Cleveland?
- Should you relocate to a retirement community where you will constantly be reassured that the world is filled with other people who have never heard of Billie Eilish?
- And perhaps most important of all, what will you actually *do* in retirement?

These are issues many of us wrestle with as we approach our golden years, particularly if we haven't managed to buy any gold, which, alas, is now at an all-time high.

Money matters

FORTUNATELY, AS A RECENT RETIREE AND CERTIFIED Financial Illiterate (CFI), I can offer some answers to many of those common financial questions you may have about retirement planning.

When should I start saving for retirement?

In general, start saving for retirement as early as possible. Set the alarm for something like 4 a.m. and check your bank account. If you can find it in the dark without bumping into the corner of the bed, then you can start saving.

And do the math. If you had started saving on a Tuesday back when you were twenty-one, say, by now you would really regret not having taken that year off backpacking across Europe when you were twenty-two. But even if you've waited to begin saving, it's never too late to start, unless it's a weekend and everything is closed.

How much should I save?

Look at it this way: If you were to put away $25 a month, each month for the next sixty-two years, including all the Februarys, would you remember where you had put all that money? Would you be able to bend down and look under the bed in case it was there? And then would you be able to bend back up?

There is a mathematical formula for figuring out how much you should save from each paycheck. It involves a complex algorithm that really is far too complex to explain.

What's a 401(k)?

A 401(k) is a workplace savings plan designed to supplement standard pension plans, which of course no longer exist. The idea is, you put in money with every paycheck and your employer puts in money with every paycheck and before you know it, your employer has gone out of business after being bought by a vulturish hedge fund.

What's a 403(b) plan?

It's two blocks down and around the corner from a 401(k) plan.

What's a Roth IRA?

Named after the novelist Philip Roth, this is a financial vehicle that lets you buy as many copies of *Portnoy's Complaint* as you'd like.

What if I'm near retirement and running out of time to save?

You can always set your clock ahead fifteen minutes and then be happily surprised that it's not as late as you thought it was. Or you can move to an earlier time zone or just wait for Daylight Savings Time.

In addition, the tax code allows for what are called "catch-up" contributions. In this way, on the day before you retire, you can finally empty that large jar in the kitchen with all the pennies you've collected and invest them into paying for dinner at the Waffle House.

Is there a certain amount of money—my "number"—that I need to have saved before I can retire?

Experts, many of whom are already retired and have nothing better to do than shame you, say to have at least seven times your salary saved by age fifty-five. By age sixty-five, you should have around ten more years and several more chronic conditions, including an inability to clear your throat.

What should I do with the money I have saved?

There are several possibilities. You could invest it in the stock market, as a hedge against inflation, which will make it sound like you know what you're doing even if you think a bear market is where you buy bears.

Just remember when you invest that past performance is no guarantee of future performance unless the past performance is really bad. And be sure, of course, to diversify your investments, putting a certain percentage of your savings under the bed while you put another percentage in the cookie jar that's on top of the fridge.

You could also buy an annuity. Annuities are complex financial instruments that can provide you with guaranteed income in retirement even if you have no idea how they work and may not be sure how they are spelled. Annuities come in three main varieties—fixed, variable, and pistachio. Be careful if you are allergic to nuts.

How can I tell the difference between a bear market and a bull market?

Bear markets are generally asleep during the winter, a period that investment analysts refer to as a market correction because the bears can correct the mistakes they made in the summer, when they told you to buy small-market honey futures.

Bull markets are generally full of bull.

When it comes to investing for retirement, how do I determine my tolerance for risk?

Ask yourself this simple question: Do you think that a convertible security is a sports car that General Motors no longer makes?

What are indexed funds?

Instead of footnotes at the bottom of each page that are really difficult to read and disrupt the flow of the narrative, indexed funds put all the relevant stuff about fees and taxes and penalties at the back of the annual report you receive from your broker. This is the report you never actually get around to reading.

What's a hedge fund, and should I put my retirement money in one?

A hedge fund is an investment partnership that is designed by rich people to make other rich people even richer. You will only be allowed to invest in a hedge fund if you already have more money than you could ever need, trust someone else with all of it, and are willing to take a blood oath in the middle of a desolate prairie.

What's the difference between tax exempt and tax deferred?

Tax planning is an essential part of any retirement investment strategy. So is having more money. While both tax exempt and tax-deferred accounts can help you minimize your tax bill in the future, making a mistake in your favor while you subtract line 72 from line 67 on your 1040 tax form is also quite effective.

What's the difference between playing the market and throwing away your money down a deep, dark hole?

Historically, throwing away your money down a deep, dark hole has only a .32 expense ratio, which, if you include dividends and redemption fees, leaves you with a vested aggregate balance of a pig in a poke. Playing the market gives you a pig without the poke.

How should I diversify my portfolio?

Buy more pokes.

If the market plummets, should I get out of stocks and go into bonds?

It would probably be better to go into plummets.

What kind of estate planning should I do?

You don't want your heirs fighting over your estate, hiring expensive lawyers, or getting enmeshed in probate and talking about you when you're not there to defend yourself. So, you need to be very committed to using up all your money and useful stuff before you go so there won't be an estate. Take that trip to Machu Picchu. Buy that enormous big screen TV. Eat out a lot.

When should I take Social Security?

You can start receiving Social Security benefits beginning at age sixty-two. But for every year you wait until you reach your full retirement age, just remember that's one more cruise or one more trip to Paris you haven't taken while you could still enjoy them.

Will Social Security be around for me when I retire?

Because there are so many of us boomers, Social Security recently has been paying out more in benefits than it receives in contributions, which means it's going to run out of money one of these days. Could be soon. So, be sure to get your requests in today; send them a nice handwritten note requesting your money and make sure to enclose a stamped, self-addressed envelope. That always works.

I am worried that I will outlive my money. What should I do?

Eat more Twinkies. You won't outlive anything.

What makes a good retirement?

Well, having that money helps, of course. Research has shown that it's much better than not having money. Seventy-eight percent of retired people with money say they wish they had 78 percent more money.

Yes, it's important to have saved for many years and to have avoided the twelve notorious retirement blunders and the seven infamous retirement mistakes. But money isn't everything, although it's a big help when you're buying stuff.

To have a successful, fulfilling retirement, you can't just lie in bed all day counting your money, no matter how attractive that is and how good a mattress you have. Sometimes you'll have to get up and go to the bathroom.

If you want to succeed at retirement, as I have, you must embrace your new status and make it meaningful. Here's how:

Learn a new skill. Learning new skills keeps a retired mind sharp. You could take up masonry or learn how to speak

French or how to sneer like the French. Personally, I have recently been practicing introductory intercranial neurosurgery. It's far more interesting than masonry, more fun than speaking French, and it has kept my mind extremely sharp, except when by mistake I take the anesthesia myself.

Learning a new skill will improve your self-confidence, help you forge new social connections, and keeps those neurons firing, even though that may give you the occasional migraine and cause the sprinklers to activate. Research has shown that being a lifelong learner can help ward off memory loss and improve cognitive abilities. And as we age, we increasingly need those cognitive abilities if the internet is down and we can't Google things.

Give back to your community. Over the years, your community has given you a lot. Now's the time to return the favor. So, get out there and clean some streets even if you do blow the leaves onto your neighbor's lawn. Frisk some dangerous-looking individuals who are just lurking around the area even if they say they are delivering the mail. Direct traffic on the nearest four-lane highway, particularly at night when motorists don't see as well and could use the help. When you're the one driving, instead of pulling over when you hear an ambulance siren behind you, plow straight ahead, leading the ambulance to where it is going. They may thank you later, or have you arrested.

Continue to challenge yourself. Just because you've gotten older doesn't mean you must shrink from mental or physical challenges. As the poet said, or should have said, a man's reach must exceed his grasp, or what's a step stool for?

Remember, you don't have to climb Everest or swim the English Channel to prove you've still got it. Instead, see if you can change the channels on your TV set without using the remote.

Try answering the phone when you don't recognize the number.

Be physically active. Make sure you get enough exercise every day, even if that means opening and closing the refrigerator door hundreds of times. Don't worry when body parts start to fall off. It's natural as we age, and some of those parts are likely not that important. For instance, did you know that the pinkie toe does pretty much nothing for you?

Do something you've never done before. It's probably too late in life to become a backup singer for Taylor Swift or write our first *bildungsroman* (German for 875 pages). But how about drinking red wine with fish? What about buying bonds when stocks go *up*? Or really how about dyeing your hair purple? Or dyeing your fish purple?

Develop a new hobby. There are lots of choices: genealogy, gardening, photography, witchcraft. Immerse yourself in the arcane details of whatever your new pastime is. Bore your friends by explaining the differences between a clematis and a petunia. Impress them with your mastery of F stops before they tell you they have an urgent call on another line.

Have a positive attitude about your future. Sometimes it's difficult to think positively, particularly when you can't find your car keys and are driving 85 on Interstate 40 or 40 on Interstate 85. Nevertheless, think of all the good things that have happened in your life and how fortunate you are that you can remember some of them. Think of how you made it through the pandemic and were able to avoid seeing your dentist for more than a year.

Then think about all the things you still can do and will do, as long as your money holds out and you don't break your hip while looking for your keys.

Get a pet. Study after study has shown that in retirement getting a pet—a dog, a cat, a Komodo dragon—can lower your blood pressure, improve your cholesterol, and enable you to have conversations with a sentient being in which no one will interrupt when you explain your theory of what's wrong with baseball today and why the new pitch clock won't fix it. Pets also provide a source of unconditional love, unless it's a cat, which doesn't give a crap.

Dogs are generally considered an appropriate pet for someone entering into or already in retirement. They are domesticated and don't like filing semi-annual performance reviews. There are many different breeds of dogs from which you can choose, including some that have evolved so much they may be able to walk themselves when it's raining outside.

Having a pet is also a great way to expand your human social circle. Strangers are more likely to introduce themselves to someone with a pet than some boomer nutso walking down the street singing 1972's "Brandy (You're a Fine Girl)," by Looking Glass.

Maintain a healthy diet. Your brain's ability to absorb and process new information is dependent on your wider physical health, which is dependent on how many utterly tasteless foods you can ingest. It's important to keep your diet balanced, alternating between foods you don't like and foods that you really hate. And always remember that tofu is not really a food and almond beverage is not a beverage.

Minimize your stress. Try not to think too much about maintaining a healthy diet, being responsible for a pet, or having a positive attitude about your future.

Be engaged. Being engaged becomes even more important as we age. Just don't tell your spouse about it.

Together forever

Actually, there's one more thing that makes a good, successful retirement and it is perhaps the most important component of all—after money, of course, and access to several premium streaming services. It's having a solid, long-term relationship, like a marriage.

But how do you stay married or just together for a long time?

The fact is, it's not easy. According to the U.S. Census Bureau, one of every two marriages ends in divorce. (The other obviously ends in Cleveland.)

As someone who has been married forever—in fact, my wife and I recently celebrated what we think is our 332nd anniversary, and it's really hard to get an appropriate card for that—we know a thing or two about marriage. As a public service, here are our marital secrets:

Secret No. 1: Have no secrets.

Admit you ate the last chocolate chip cookie. Confess that you were the one who left the toilet seat up. Again. Willingly share that for the last seventeen years you have been an undercover North Korean spy.

Secret No. 2: Lower your expectations.

It's important to remember that marriage isn't always perfect. Sometimes there will be bumps in the road and the coffee will spill in your lap because *someone* forgot to put the cover on the travel mug correctly, although we're not naming names here. So, when there are bumps along the road, remember they are almost always your partner's fault because you would have taken a different road, probably the interstate.

Secret No. 3: Happily-ever-after doesn't mean life together will be a fairy tale.

Instead of a fairy tale, sometimes married life will be a collection of oblique *New Yorker* short stories where there are no "he saids" and "she saids," and you can't tell which partner in the marriage is speaking and which one isn't listening. Sometimes, married life will be a limerick, usually one ending in a naughty word. From time to time, married life will seem like a nineteenth-century Russian novel where everyone is named Goncharov or Carolnikov and you can't tell what chapter you are in but still have eight hundred more pages to read.

Secret No. 4: Don't hold a grudge.

But keep it nearby if someone asks you to do the dishes when you'd prefer to mindlessly scroll through Facebook. Then you can pick it up and say, sorry, I can't, I'm holding a grudge from the last time you asked me and so my hands are full.

Secret No. 5: Never go to bed angry.

This may mean unfortunately that you have to avoid sleeping for several weeks. During this time, drink a lot of coffee and pop some energy shots. If you get really tired, read a good Russian novel with characters named Goncharov or Carolnikov. You won't sleep, but at least your eyes will glaze over.

Secret No. 6: Communication is important.

At breakfast, while sitting directly across the table from each other, be sure to send your partner a text. Check to make sure you're both skimming similar Twitter feeds. Snapchat with him or her while in bed. Post to each other's Instagram while you're driving together to pick up the kids or grandkids.

Secret No. 7: Show respect to your partner by paying attention.

Excuse me, what was that secret? Could you repeat it? Could you repeat the others, too?

You've got (to have) a friend

I KNOW WHAT SOME OF YOU ARE THINKING: WHAT IF I don't have a partner from whom I can keep secrets?

For some of us, it's true—our partner has passed away or worse, moved to Boca Raton. And a few of us have never had a true partner and have spent much of our recent adult life arguing with customer service representatives. .

Not only do some of us not have partners, many of us no longer have many friends. Long gone are the days when we'd all leave the office together and stop somewhere to get a drink and someone would have too much to drink and fall off the bar stool. Long gone are the days where we'd all hang out at the coffee shop or go to the movies together or spend hours trying to decide if we should all hang out at the coffee shop or go to the movies together.

For one thing, who wants to go to the coffee shop now when there's a long line of latte-drinking poseurs there and you've already spent a fortune on buying your own fair-trade, single-origin certified Arabica coffee beans? And who wants to go to the movies when you subscribe to nine different streaming channels and still would prefer to watch black-and-white reruns of *The Life and Legend of Wyatt Earp* on a cable channel no one's ever heard of?

Plus, many of the old gang, our old friends, no longer live nearby and anyway only want to know if you have been able to figure out the new Medicare guidelines. Also, the kids are now far away and preoccupied with their own kids and a completely different set of streaming channels. Meanwhile, the neighbors are cooking meth in their basements and the friends we made at school or at work or down at the local bar are all busy checking their timelines on Facebook, and the local bar is now a Starbucks full of baristas with purple hair.

(I should point out here that I am fortunate in that I do still have a few friends. We meet regularly for lunches and spend most of our time trying to answer last night's Final Jeopardy question. Unfortunately, the category frequently is baroque music or extinct birds and none of us has a clue. Plus, we often forget to put our answers in the form of questions.)

Not everyone, I understand, is as fortunate as I am. Many of us feel alone and we are not alone in feeling alone. According to research done by researchers who have been locked in caves and able to delve deeply into datasets because their phones rarely ping, that sense of isolation is pretty common when we get to a certain age. It's a situation that undoubtedly was exacerbated by the pandemic, leaving many boomers stuck at home by ourselves, spending most of our waking hours chatting with Alexa and Siri about Tony Orlando and Dawn.

This sense of isolation and lack of social connectedness can be harmful to our physical and mental health and ultimately lead to an increased risk of dementia, heart disease, and an inability to correctly identify kohlrabi. Social connection and interaction make us feel better, heighten our self-esteem, and actually lower our blood pressure while reducing the risk of cognitive decline. Plus, those who are socially connected are 73 percent less likely to want to watch episodes of *Family Feud*.

But how do you get connected if you're just sitting around all day waiting for the clothes washer beep signaling the end of the spin cycle and worrying that you're just sitting around all day waiting for the clothes washer beep signaling the end of the spin cycle?

I have some suggestions:

Join a book club. This will enable you to get together once a month with a sociable group of people who also aren't sure how to correctly operate a Kindle. For an hour or so, you'll spend time discussing the last book you've read and how the movie was better. Then, you'll spend the next hour or so arguing about the next book you should all read before ultimately agreeing on a book nobody likes and nobody will finish in time for the next book club meeting. Then you will all start yawning because it's almost nine o'clock and getting near bedtime.

Enroll in a class. Continuing education is not just important for your cognitive health and keeping your mind sharp; it's also an opportunity to meet other like-minded people with curious minds even if some might have purple hair and a few have no hair at all.

For instance, go take a calculus class at a local university or community college near you. You will not understand a single word spoken by the instructor, of course, but you can be assured that none of your younger classmates will either because, hey, it's calculus. However, they are likely to take you under their wing and anoint you as their mascot and ask you to pledge Beta Kappa Feta, one of the cheesiest fraternities.

Sign up for an online dating service if you're really single. First, carefully build your online dating profile, being sure to use a photo taken back when your hair was still black and your stomach still flat, if it ever was. (But probably don't use the one where you're wearing the bright green polyester leisure suit.)

In your bio, mention your Olympic gold medal and your Purple Heart. And just remember that if you feel slightly awkward about your embellishments, the individuals you meet online will almost assuredly not really look like the picture they used and also may not have won multiple Nobel Peace Prizes.

Join a travel group. With work not a factor and family not nearby, it's time to travel! See Paris with others who haven't figured out euros and think the French are snobby by insisting on speaking French! Visit Venice with people who can't hold their Chianti! Voyage to the far reaches of the earth along with other intrepid voyagers who will spend most of the communal breakfast making sure they've taken all their pills!

Attend a protest. Political activism is a great way to meet people with similar views and commitments in your area. Plus, there's a serious sense of camaraderie at protests and you'll have lots of time to talk and get to know fellow protestors while waiting to be bailed out by your kids. In addition, you may finally be able to use some of the signs you proudly if inexplicably saved in the back of the upstairs closet from that 1974 antiwar march.

Get a dog. As noted earlier, dogs are an appropriate pet for someone who is retired. But, in addition, having a dog is also a good way to make new friends.

You have to walk a dog, which means you will have to get out of the house and will likely come in contact with other people out walking who will admire your dog's coat, ask you about the dog's breed, the age of the dog, and why the hell are you letting it poop on their lawn?

You also will meet other people out walking their dogs and who are equally pissed off that they had to go out in the rain and sleet twice that day for that mutt their kids *promised* they would be responsible for and take care of. And if you have a snarling, aggressive dog that bites complete strangers, that's always a good conversation starter that may lead to a lasting friendship or at least a long-running legal case.

Strike up a conversation with a stranger. When you're out for a walk and get mugged, see if the mugger is interested in traveling or maybe joining a book club.

Frequently Asked Questions

Now that you have almost reached the end of this book, it's possible you still have some questions about how to become a better boomer. Fortunately, I still have some answers.

Why do you say "frequently asked questions" rather than FAQs?

This is not a website or a long text message or a Facebook post. It is a book, something we used to read before we discovered podcasts. Also, I believe, IMHO, acronyms are ruining modern conversation. OTOH, I could be wrong, but that's my POV.

How can a reader get the most out of the book and become a better boomer?

For full appreciation, sit back in your best recliner, take a deep breath, gently close your eyes and promise to never utter the word *influencer*. It's also good if you still believe that

Drake is a coffee cake. Plus, you need to be reasonably conversant with what was considered pop culture in 1965 even if you were barely alive in 1965 and also can't remember what happened on Tuesday.

Have any subjects been harmed in the construction of this book?

No experimentation has been allowed in these pages, except, occasionally, I may have tried to see how one of my jokes went down with my wife and asked if she thought something was funny. Most of the time, she didn't. Only rarely did she complain of acute abdominal pain caused by excessive chuckling.

Has this book been tested on animals?

Yes, and they laughed at us. Well, the chimps did, but they laugh at everything.

Where do you get your ideas for the book?

Being a boomer takes years of practice. It's almost as if you have to have been born more than half a century ago. Then, once you have reached the age where, technically speaking, your bones crack when you get up from a chair, you then begin to carefully cultivate and prune random thoughts and complaints and the occasional kvetch.

You may need to regularly add some manure if the ideas are not yet ripe and you are regular. (A few ideas, unfortunately, only blossom during idea harvest season.)

How do you know if something is funny?

If someone laughs, unless it's my wife, that's a good sign. If she laughs, then I know I've probably stolen the joke from someone. Fortunately, neither of us remembers from whom.

Are reservations needed?

The book is first-come, first-served. But reservations are always a good idea, particularly if you want to gain access to the good paragraphs first.

Is the book hypoallergenic?

We believe it is, although since we're not certain if hypoallergenic means too allergic or not allergic enough, we can't be sure.

Is special training needed to become a humor writer?

Not really, although it does help if you've taken doctoral-level courses in puns and been inducted into the Légion d'Honneur for knowing how to juggle metaphors and where to put apostrophes.

How can I send multiple texts through this book? Can you view live video streaming with this book? Is the book on Netflix? How can I fix syncing problems? Does the book have a Quad HD Super AMOLED display?

I think you may have confused this book with the Samsung X2500 GS 476-3 Rocket-Launched Pebble Blue model. It's a fairly common mistake.

When will the podcast drop?

Unfortunately, there is, at this time, no podcast of this book. There is also no YA version, nor Broadway musical, *Cliff's Notes* guide, novelization, nor upcoming television series. We continue to work on the Sunday morning cartoon and TikTok dance tie-in, but for the moment, there is only this book, and, of course, its accompanying Young Thug soundtrack album.

How often does a question have to be asked before it can be considered frequently asked?

At least twice.

How often does a question have to be asked before it can be considered frequently asked?

Do you use algorithms in figuring out what topics will be most appealing to boomer readers and sell them to advertisers?

We would, if we truly knew we have spelled algorithm correctly. Also, we're not completely sure if it's different from logarithm.

By the way, if you know any advertisers who would be interested, please tell us how to get in touch with them.

Are there any special apps for the book?

We are in the process of developing special apps for the book that would allow the reader to quickly search for all Tommy James and the Shondells references and also to find nearby restaurants that don't use the term "locally grown" on their menus.

Is an unlimited data plan offered with the book?

Since there is very little data offered with the book, at this time we're offering only limited data plans. Everybody just gets one date. For instance, I have taken April 25. It's my birthday.

When you are writing a book, do you have a deadline?

Yes. It's now.

What is the most important quality in a humor book?

Brevity.

In Closing

You can build a better boomer, but even the better boomer better beware. There is, unfortunately, a limit to how much better we can become.

Yes, after much study, we can occasionally identify some artisanal cheeses and a few Brooklyn-based craft beers. With practice, we frequently can remember to take our keys *and* our glasses when we leave the house. If we concentrate, we may finally figure out how to navigate a patient portal, whether on our desktop, laptop, tablet, smartphone or, most likely, by calling our kids and pleading for help.

We now realize, most of all, that it's a good idea to start planning for retirement while in preschool, and we know about the critical importance of getting enough sleep, regular exercise, eating well, updating our technology regularly, and being socially engaged, even if we do none of that and would prefer to watch old episodes of *Taxi*.

Yet despite all our efforts and our newly acquired knowledge, we persist in getting older, if we're lucky, and appear to be floating further away from the current zeitgeist. Assuming we know what a zeitgeist is and are certain it's not the name of a new subreddit.

That is, some of us continue to dwell in the past and not remember the passwords. When our children and grandchildren talk about crypto, we may continue to think we hear them discussing Crisco, the all-vegetable shortening.

In fact, although we still may want to think the world revolves around our boomer generation, we must ultimately acknowledge that we continue to be unable to identify a single member of BTS. (It's a boy band, from Korea.)

Consequently, we must recognize there's nothing more to be done here. Our work is finished and we are going to have to shut down this book now.

Very soon, the adverbs will be leaving their cubicles. Conjunctions will be walking off the assembly line. Prepositions will be logging out of their workstations.

All but essential workers—those who continue to protect the book against really dumb grammatical errors and the dedicated line workers who operate the spell-check machine—have been furloughed. In the spirit of boomerdom, they have retired.

Following this shutdown, only extremely crucial sentences and some useful paraphrases will be allowed into this space. Key operations, such as clever plays on words and intricate puns, will be suspended until further notice.

We understand that this closure will cause significant

upheaval in the lives of those boomers who have grown to depend on clever parodies, age-appropriate cultural references and insightful kvetching to get them through another hard day of trying to figure out what to do with their old record albums. We are sympathetic to those who relied on our witty jabs to help them forget that the end of the Vietnam War is now about as long ago as the end of World War I was during the Vietnam War. We identify with all those who just want to skim some easy-to-read pages between sets of more pickleball and put off trying to decipher the video instruction manual for the new high-tech kitchen blender.

But we really do need to get in our nap, so we leave you, then, with one pivotal question: Can an illustrious demographic cohort, which persevered through eight-track tape players, high-intensity interval free-range SoulCycle and pet rocks, continue its fight against creeping kombucha, technospeak, and dangling dongles?

Honestly, we have no idea, but we thank you for your attention and also for your willingness to give us a good review on Amazon.

Acknowledgments

Without the help of all those working behind the scenes and several who worked in front of the scenes and those brave few who dared to work on the slippery sides of the scenes, this book would not have been possible. Of course, then again, it might have been better.

First of all, I'd like to acknowledge my wife, Carol, who insisted I acknowledge her first. She also convinced me to call this section of the book my "Acknowledgments" rather than the more listless Chapter 11, particularly since that was already taken and also because it might make readers think I was declaring bankruptcy. She also helped me compile all these acknowledgments, using her unsurpassed threatening skills, and made sure her name would come first even if I did it alphabetically.

I'd also like here to thank my children, Paul and Nora, for being my children and rarely reminding me of that time in the

Denver airport when I lost my mind during that five-hour delay and told the ticket agent I would never ever again mention the Denver airport in any of my acknowledgments.

Thanks, too, to the ticket agent, without whom this anger would have gone away years ago but has stayed boiling within me to fuel my vicious but rivetingly amusing attacks on airports.

I'd also like to thank my butcher, Cliff, for his hamburger patties and his steadfast commitment to the 80-20 fat ratio. And I can't forget the work of my plumber, Hal, who was able to plumb the depths of my comic despair over growing older while never forgetting that the kitchen trash masher still wasn't working.

I would not have gotten to this point without my faithful translators, the ones in Germany and France, Estonia and Kazakhstan, Malta, and Jersey City. They have been able to evocatively convey the essence of this book, the distillation of the poetry, even if they didn't fully understand several of the words I was using, many of the obscure 1960s cultural references, and believed this book needed more umlauts.

Let me take a moment here to single out my agent, Van Riper-Stephens-Cramer, for his tireless refusal to take no for an answer even when the answer was no.

I also owe a great debt to those who have come before me: Dickens, Proust, Turgenev, and the other kids in my multicultural preschool class at Miss Peacock's, who helped me line up in size places.

I am greatly appreciative of the efforts of my friends Rob, Marty, Dick, Frank, and Mitch (not to be confused with editors Mitch, Frank, Dick, Marty, and Rob), who have read different parts of this manuscript and who all agreed emphatically that I should become a butcher.

And, of course, I would be remiss if I didn't mention Miss Bave, my first-grade teacher, who taught me everything I know about macro-economic theory.

Finally, my greatest thanks of all go to my imaginary dog Pamplemousse, for chewing up the first version of these acknowledgments.

About the Author

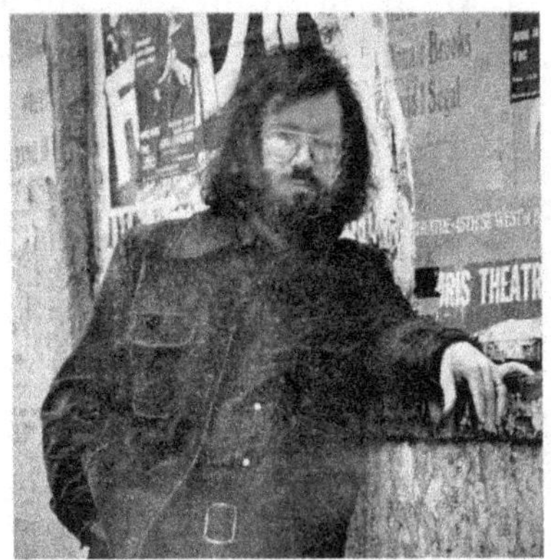

Then

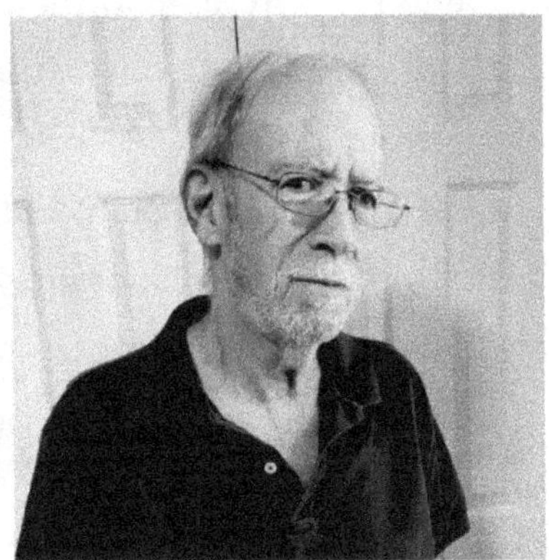

Now

NEIL OFFEN IS THE INTERNATIONALLY BESTSELLING author of the international bestsellers *The Getting Fat and Staying Fat Diet* and *The Insider's Guide to Cultivating Insomnia*. He is, as well, the man behind several critically acclaimed supermarket shopping lists.

Lauded as "that guy" by *The New York Times* and hailed as "him," by National Public Radio, Offen has been published in a variety of formats, including pen, crayon. chalk and, once, under duress, his wife's eyebrow pencil.

He has received many honors, beginning with the bronze medal in his fourth-grade spelling bee contest, which he definitely would have won if not for the word *surprize*, and has been named "Un Homme Très Etrange," by the French government, the highest honor it can bestow on someone who doesn't know how to pronounce ratatouille.

Offen comes from Modest Means, a small town south of Sheboygan, WI. He would have grown up in a log cabin if his family had been able to carry more logs onto the subway. Although his parents had planned on his pursuing a career as a nuclear physicist, even if they had no idea what that was, Offen instead showed his preference for using words, frequently coming in a close second in family Scrabble games. He would have even won one game, too, if he had only known how to use the magic cube to spell physicist.

Offen began his writing career early, writing notes home from summer camp pleading with his parents to please get him out of there before the Junior Buckskins would be attempting the zip line over the lake on Thursday.

While in school, he forged ahead in his writing career, devoting himself to the intellectually challenging pursuit of writing limericks when he should have been paying attention in math class. He ultimately gave up that career when he ran out of acceptable rhymes for limericks that began, "There once was a man from Nantucket."

A master of multiple styles of writing, Offen has dipped his pen in journalism, poetry, fiction, nonfiction, IOUs, and absolute lying. An early adopter of the new digital technology to enhance his writing, he has managed to inadvertently delete important things he has written from his desktop, his laptop, his iPad, and his iPhone.

His works, particularly his emails and some of his texts, are in the permanent collection of his friends Dick, Marty, Mitch, Frank, and Richard, mainly because they are old and none of them is quite sure yet how to permanently delete items from a Gmail inbox.

Offen has written for the neighborhood listserv, frequently asking for recommendations for reliable handymen, and contributed as well to birthday cards for most members of his immediate family.

He lives in Carrboro, North Carolina, but likes to imagine he's still in the south of France, where the wine is cheaper, which is why he always says *bonjour* to the mailman and occasionally to the next-door neighbors. The neighbors have occasionally tried to have him committed, but the authorities no longer respond to their hysterical calls.

Offen lives with his wife and three imaginary dogs, because they could never get a real one since he's allergic. His two real children have never forgiven him for that.

Index

Aches. *See* pains, 1–173; in knees, left 26–94, right 18–102; both at same time, 74–76; lower back, *see* just above right hip; hips, *see* just below achy back; excruciating, 7, 23, 114; bearable with extra alcohol, 37; annoying, 4, 107; reasons to nevertheless avoid seeing a doctor, 14, 26–31, 86, 111.

Aging, 2, 4, 6, 11, 25, 26–174; inevitability, 2, 4, 6, 8, who do we appreciate? relationship to getting older, 4, 27, 93–94; alternatives to: cremation, 6; forming new garage band, 51; buying a Porsche, 66; opening TikTok account, 104; lying about your age, 143. *See* also obsession with youth, 100, and Botox, 49, Viagra, 56, Grecian Formula, 88, and Instagram, 113.

Cruise, Tom. *See Top Gun*, definitely *The Firm*, maybe *Minority Report*. Definitely don't *see Eyes Wide Shut*.

Dementia, 23, 23, 23, 23, 23, 23; not the same as regular forgetfulness, 29, 68; still worried though, 30, 69; benefits of, line 3, last two words..

Diet: foods to avoid, 38–99; foods to eat, 40–43.04; superfoods, 19–22; good-enough foods, 6–78; bad foods but they really taste good, 30–74; losing weight, 188–35=153.

Doohickey. *See* whatchamacallit, 116.

Drugs, 7, 57, 96, hike; dangers of, 44–98; benefits of, 2–61, 79, 104; forgetting to get refills, 87; side effects, *see* Tractors, do not operate, 45–46.

Exercise, 14, 19-22, 102, 122-59; worse than colonoscopy prep, 88-90; better than doing taxes, 35-38; excuses to use to abstain from, 91-95; embarrassing dangers of, including dumbbell drops, 5, 31, 114-125; overuse injuries from 26-28, 99-104, 125; dangers of watching home improvement shows while on treadmill, 76-81.

Insurance, health: Medicare, 98, 100, 102-05; Advantage plans, 105-07; Disadvantage plans, 108–09; No advantage plans, 109-10.

iPhone. *See* landline, if you still can.

Pains. *See* aches, 173–1 (Hebrew version); complaints about, 46–87; living with, 92–144; living without, 2. *Also see* agonizing, excruciating, throbbing, and that burning sensation you get after eating too much pizza for breakfast, 118.

Retirement: Planning for 99–105; saving for 114–129; wasting 144–169; enjoyment of wasting, 170–175; watching too much Weather Channel, 202.

Technology: Importance of, 33–35, 48, 71, 89–102;

aggravations from, 33–35, 48, 71, 89–102; *see* dongle, router, update, RAM, ROM, thingamajig.

Youth: Wasted on young, 109.

ZIP codes: 27516, 84480, 11203, 25143.

Printed in the USA
CPSIA information can be obtained
at www.ICGtesting.com
LVHW051707021223
765402LV00002B/243